Sustainable Development Goals Series

The Sustainable Development Goals Series is Springer Nature's inaugural cross-imprint book series that addresses and supports the United Nations' seventeen Sustainable Development Goals. The series fosters comprehensive research focused on these global targets and endeavors to address some of society's grand challenges. The SDGs are inherently multidisciplinary, and they bring people working across different fields together toward a common goal. In this spirit, the Sustainable Development Goals series is the first at Springer Nature to publish books under both the Springer and Palgrave Macmillan imprints, bringing the strengths of our imprints together.

The Sustainable Development Goals Series is organized into eighteen subseries: one subseries based around each of the seventeen respective Sustainable Development Goals, and an eighteenth subseries, "Connecting the Goals," which serves as a home for volumes addressing multiple goals or studying the SDGs as a whole. Each subseries is guided by an expert Subseries Advisor with years or decades of experience studying and addressing core components of their respective SDG.

The SDG Series has a remit as broad as the SDGs themselves, and contributions are welcome from scientists, academics, policymakers, and researchers working in fields related to any of the seventeen goals. If you are interested in contributing a monograph or curated volume to the series, please contact the Publishers: Zachary Romano [Springer; zachary.romano@springer.com] and Rachael Ballard [Palgrave Macmillan; rachael.ballard@palgrave.com].

More information about this series at
http://www.palgrave.com/gp/series/15486

Pauline B. Thompson · Kerry Taylor

A Cultural Safety Approach to Health Psychology

palgrave
macmillan

Pauline B. Thompson
Psychology
Pennsylvania State University
Media, PA, USA

Kerry Taylor
College of Medicine and Public Health
Flinders University
Adelaide, SA, Australia

ISSN 2523-3084   ISSN 2523-3092 (electronic)
Sustainable Development Goals Series
ISBN 978-3-030-76848-5   ISBN 978-3-030-76849-2 (eBook)
https://doi.org/10.1007/978-3-030-76849-2

© The Editor(s) (if applicable) and The Author(s), under exclusive license to Springer Nature Switzerland AG 2021
Color wheel and icons: From https://www.un.org/sustainabledevelopment/, Copyright © 2020 United Nations. Used with the permission of the United Nations.
This work is subject to copyright. All rights are solely and exclusively licensed by the Publisher, whether the whole or part of the material is concerned, specifically the rights of translation, reprinting, reuse of illustrations, recitation, broadcasting, reproduction on microfilms or in any other physical way, and transmission or information storage and retrieval, electronic adaptation, computer software, or by similar or dissimilar methodology now known or hereafter developed.
The use of general descriptive names, registered names, trademarks, service marks, etc. in this publication does not imply, even in the absence of a specific statement, that such names are exempt from the relevant protective laws and regulations and therefore free for general use.
The publisher, the authors and the editors are safe to assume that the advice and information in this book are believed to be true and accurate at the date of publication. Neither the publisher nor the authors or the editors give a warranty, expressed or implied, with respect to the material contained herein or for any errors or omissions that may have been made. The publisher remains neutral with regard to jurisdictional claims in published maps and institutional affiliations.

Cover illustration: Christian Ohde/Alamy Stock Photo

Disclaimer: The content of this publication has not been approved by the United Nations and does not reflect the views of the United Nations or its officials or Member States.

This Palgrave Macmillan imprint is published by the registered company Springer Nature Switzerland AG
The registered company address is: Gewerbestrasse 11, 6330 Cham, Switzerland

Preface

Welcome to this book, *A Cultural Safety Approach to Health Psychology*.

We begin by acknowledging the Indigenous Peoples across the globe and that we respect their relationships with their Lands. We acknowledge the complex histories of displacement, enslavement, genocide and assimilation through colonization that have contributed, and continue to contribute, to our current circumstances. This book is one offering to repairing relationships. Throughout are examples of healing approaches that contend with the ongoing effects of colonialism. Our hope is that psychologists, health and human services practitioners, and researchers will be inspired to maintain and enhance their relationships with Indigenous communities and other communities who have been or continue to be harmed through colonialism. We hope that readers will seek to initiate those relationships in their own communities and through their work.

Before you read on, could we please ask you to remove your culture at the door? Strange request? An impossible request. Culture is not something that can be removed like a pair of shoes. It can be changed, adapted, influenced and more, but culture in whatever form, comes with us, which is why it is such a crucial consideration for working in culturally diverse fields relevant to health psychology such as health and human services. Importantly, within the concept of cultural safety, culture is defined in a broader sense, to relate to more than race or ethnicity, making the applicability of this approach relevant to any setting. Culture and cultural difference can be considered in terms of any potential point of distinction.

Aimed at educating both lower and upper-level undergraduate psychology students, we apply the concept of cultural safety to health and human services in the U.S. context. Whether or not students go on to pursue further degrees, many of them will go on to work in health and human services, education, or other professional fields requiring interactions with people that will benefit from a culturally safe approach. In this book, we have focused on health and human services and have used this phrase throughout. We encourage users/readers to broaden the applicability of this material to areas such as education, criminal justice, or other fields.

Educating health and human service professionals is an incredibly important, as well as daunting task in a current climate that is often ambivalent at least and hostile at worst. Health, social and human service professionals are at the forefront of interactions with people who may be different to themselves in terms of race, ethnicity, gender, sexuality, age, religion, migration status, geographic location, class and poverty, and abilities. These interactions can influence health and social outcomes and contribute positively or negatively to overall health disparities. We have aimed to provide a range of examples throughout but, because the basis of cultural safety is to acknowledge the enduring harmful effects of colonialism, many of our examples and discussions relate to Native and Black Americans.

There are good reasons for focusing our attention to cultural safety for professional work in health and human services. Cultural discordance, or a difference in background between professionals and their clients, has been shown to have an impact on the care provided and how it is received. This is not necessarily a conscious act, which is all the more reason to focus our attention on the cultural safety of professional care encounters.

Through case studies, discussions, reflections and critiques of social issues in the United States today, this book offers a starting point—for undergraduate students in applied disciplines such as psychology, counselling, social work, health care, nursing, and family studies who require an introduction to the area—for learning about cultural safety. The material covered has evolved from extensive research and teaching in health, culture, diversity, Indigeneity and racism in three countries. The book focuses on a cultural safety approach, the main model used in health education in New Zealand, Australia and Canada and is emerging in the U.S. While intended as an introduction, the issues and ideas can and should be adapted to suit local settings. Using this book for education purposes requires consultation with local communities about the appropriateness and relevance of the content in their area. Local adaptation of the discussions and information is expected and required. The social model of health is thoroughly applied throughout with considerations for health behaviors and concerns at the individual, family, community, and wider political, cultural and social levels. A decolonizing approach woven throughout, draws the reader's attention to how worldviews and culture influence health care provision and behaviors and our interpretation of information.

The thirteen chapters include:

1. *Introduction and Terminology* presents an overview to this book and the concept of cultural safety as a preferred way of working as professionals and considers terminology to use when working in cultural contexts. Establishing the correct terminology is like a respectful introduction where you tell someone your name and how you would like to be addressed. We also begin to explore the need to decolonize our professional practice.
2. *Culture-focused Frameworks for Service Delivery* includes a comparative analysis of various approaches to health care such as cultural awareness, cultural sensitivity, cultural competence, cultural humility and cultural responsiveness, to understanding and addressing cultural issues and considerations from a professional practice standpoint.
3. *Cultural Safety* describes the concept of cultural safety and the rationale for its preferred use as an underpinning philosophy and the

guiding principles for practice. In this chapter, the practice principles of cultural safety are discussed and include reflection on practice; the importance of communication and asking questions; consideration of power differentials; being mindful of how colonization impacts practice; racism and discrimination awareness; and ensuring that professionals do not diminish, demean or disempower others through their interactions.

4. *Models of Health and Well-Being* presents a conceptual background to thinking about health, mental health and well-being. The majority of health and human service professionals in the U.S. subscribe to a biomedical model. This chapter considers various models and definitions of health and how they fit within the context of diverse and complex client care.

5. In *History Taking*, we discuss the importance of understanding history in healthcare and human services work. We address how historical relationships, policies and events relate to health and wellbeing and to health and social disparities in the U.S. today. This chapter presents descriptions of past practices that are not only known to be unethical by any standard but proven to have had a detrimental effect on the health and well-being of subsequent generations.

6. *Consuming Research* discusses research from the perspective of professionals as critical consumers of research and provides readers with tips and skills for assessing research quality and understanding the implications of research findings. We discuss logic systems and worldviews as they relate to creating, developing, and interpreting research through the lens of cultural safety. Research methods and processes, including community based participatory research, will be explored in relation to culturally safe principles. The role of unethical research in our past in contributing to distrust of health care is examined along with research ethics today.

7. *Determinants of Health* explores the influences on health beyond an individual's biological or behavioral health. These influences include education, poverty, employment, and housing. Importantly, all of these influences are also determined by politics, racism, and discrimination. Readers will be encouraged to reflect on their own cultures

and identities and the potential impact on others; to identify examples of systemic bias, institutional and individual racism and discrimination; and to analyze and discuss determinants of health.
8. In *Stats and Maps* we explore various sources of information that can be helpful to our learning and understanding about culture and diversity. We examine the roles of epidemiology and human geography and discuss some of the limitations of pitfalls of large-scale data. We explore some of the myths and stereotyped ideas that can interfere with culturally safe practice and attempt to counter some of the misconceptions with an overview of the demographic and health statistics. We also consider the use of maps as valuable sources of information.
9. *Special Interest and Priority Areas* explores areas of special interest in the U.S., including maternal and child health, chronic and infectious disease, substance abuse, mental health issues, disability and aging. It offers rationales for giving attention to certain groups and issues and asks students to consider what issues are relevant in their local settings. This chapter focuses on just some of the current major health issues faced in the U.S. and the potential role of professionals in addressing these in a culturally safe manner. It is not possible to look at all major health concerns, so we review a selection of the key national priorities.
10. *Capacity and Resilience* discusses these concepts that contrast with the tendency of governments and others to take a deficits approach rather than focusing on strengths. A cultural safety approach requires a reorientation—from positioning certain populations as problematic to focusing on strengths, capacity and resilience. Such a reorientation also fits well with the principles of primary health care (PHC) and community psychology. This chapter explores the potential for success in health and social outcomes that can be achieved from a simple change in view, while also maintaining the stance that improvement in health of all sectors of the community is everyone's responsibility.
11. *Intercultural Communication* presents a range of case studies related to healthcare communications. Conflicting worldviews and miscommunication are major challenges when professionals differ in cultural

and linguistic background from the clients in their care. This chapter provides an opportunity to examine intercultural interactions in various practice settings, as well as exploring what it means to 'decolonize' practice and looks at health literacy as both an individual and organizational responsibility.

12. *Comparable Contexts* looks briefly at the experiences of colonization and race relations in Canada, New Zealand and Australia and the impacts on health and wellbeing. Colonization affected Indigenous and other populations all around the world, both in its impact through 'settlements' and through the enslavement, forced removal and other efforts that led to the forced relocation of people. While there are many similarities in the effects of colonization in various countries, there are also some important differences that can help us to understand what contributes to these impacts and how to move forward. This will provide a barometer for evaluating our progress in promoting health equity for Indigenous Peoples and other groups harmed through colonialism.

13. *Reflection as a Tool of Culturally Safe Practice* describes this key component of culturally safe practice and provides some strategies for reflection on previously held assumptions, beliefs and attitudes. Reflection is a powerful tool for learning, development and growth. Through reflection, in and on practice, health and human service professionals have an opportunity to examine their interactions with the goal of providing culturally safe and effective care. Reflection is applied to help health and human service professionals to decolonize and move toward culturally safe practice. Finally, we examine the relevance of this topic to professional practice, and the transferability of reflective practice that is regardful in any setting.

What to Expect and What Not to Expect

Each chapter may be read as a standalone, however, we recommend working through the text as much as possible from beginning to end, as content is built upon and revisited throughout. The authors aim to model the principles of cultural safety that are the focus of this book. To this end, we have approached this work as a conversation in which readers are invited to engage, rather than a uni-directional academic pronouncement. The language is intentionally accessible. We provide opportunities for reflection and critical thinking throughout. We model the decolonizing approach through the use of stories, poems, and conversations rather than emphasizing academic narrative and Western knowledge. We provide guidance on where to look for more information, and ways to see and understand information through a lens of cultural safety.

This is a book about health and social issues. The topics at times are confronting or difficult. Readers should be aware of this and engage in self-care as appropriate and take the time to reflect on reactions to material.

What we will not be doing is presenting a case by case of each cultural group's supposed health or social issues. We will not provide a checklist of what people belonging to specific cultures or population groups are expected to need in health or human services, based on stereotyped views or biased information. Thus, we will not perpetuate Western tendencies to categorize and label, nor do we suggest specific practices that will 'fix' clients or persons receiving care or services.

Each chapter presents case studies and scenarios to illustrate key learnings. Critical thinking questions are designed to help unpack the points demonstrated. Importantly, throughout, readers are asked to link their learning and investigations to their local settings. The text stems from the co-authors' previous work in the field of cultural safety education in Australian Indigenous health but seeks to demonstrate the transferability of cultural safety as a concept with great relevance and potential for addressing health and social disparities in the U.S.

We also want to declare that we, the authors, are two White women, one American and one Australian. Some may (and some have) questioned how culturally safe it is to have two women of relative privilege present material such as this. We have asked ourselves the same question, but always return to the belief that cultural safety is everybody's responsibility, and everybody's right to expect in their experiences of health and human services. This is our opportunity to practice one of the essential elements of cultural safety—that of reflecting on our own cultures and examining how these might contribute to diminishing, demeaning or disempowering other cultural groups. We also both share personal as well as professional experiences of intercultural relationships and being members of cultural minorities ourselves, in specific aspects of our lives, that have challenged our thinking and ways of being in the world. Between us, as authors, we identify as women, veteran, who identify as part of the broader LGBTQ community, in interracial relationships, and with various disabilities and challenges from traumatic experiences of our own. Between us we are mothers, step-mother, grandmother or caregivers to 16 children with various disabilities, who identify as parts of the LGBTQ communities, who are White, Black, Indigenous, and migrants.

We believe there is nothing written like this for U.S. psychology and health and human service students, insofar as we have tried to decolonize our own Western academic didactic style of writing to model another cultural safety principle—of engaging in dialogue. The readers are invited to share and reflect on personal and local contexts and we invite readers to take the ideas further, to unpack and critique them and hopefully, find value in developing culturally safe ways of working as psychology and health and human services professionals.

Media, PA, USA	Pauline B. Thompson
Adelaide, Australia	Kerry Taylor

Acknowledgments

Acknowledgments for Pauline B. Thompson

In the spirit of healing, I'd like to acknowledge the traditional peoples of the lands that I call home, the Lenni Lenape, and acknowledge all who have been displaced or harmed through genocide, enslavement, or assimilation. May our work serve as our contribution to healing the harms and preventing new ones. I thank my children for their support, many conversations and sharing with me their lives and their own experiences that have helped me to grow and appreciate even more the critical importance of this work. I thank my husband, Ulysses, for opening the doors for me to see a whole new world and deepening my compassion and faith.

Thank you, Kerry, for agreeing to do this with me…again. You're the best co-author, and I am truly grateful for our friendship as well as our working relationship. I'd say we're getting pretty good at this!

Acknowledgments for Kerry Taylor

I want to acknowledge that I am living and working on lands never ceded, and pay my respects to the traditional owners, past, present and continuing, of the country I call home, Australia. The body of knowledge I have drawn upon for this work, has been developed over some forty-plus years, working in areas of cultural diversity, health and education. I thank my many teachers who have shared their insights and knowledges with me. I thank my family, Vick and Nungarrayi—the greatest life teacher of all; Kelly and Phillipus families, and friends and colleagues over many years,—too many to list, but who have helped shape my understandings presented in this text.

Importantly, I want to acknowledge my friend and co-author, Pauline, for the opportunity and invitation to collaborate on what I hope will be a welcome contribution to the field of cultural safety. It was a daunting prospect to focus our attention on such an extraordinarily complex country as the United States, but also an exciting one. We always manage to add a few more grey hairs to the collection, and undertaking this work during a global pandemic, certainly added another layer, but it also brought home the importance of this work, which we both believe has the greatest potential to improve health outcomes in any setting. We also managed some laughs—maybe nervous laughter—along the way. Thank you again, Pauline.

From both Kerry and Pauline: We would like to thank the team at Palgrave Macmillan for their support throughout this project. We would also like to acknowledge the many helpful comments and feedback from both formal and informal reviewers.

Praise for *A Cultural Safety Approach to Health Psychology*

"This book is an invaluable resource for psychology students that puts cultural safety at the forefront of physical and mental health and facilitates thinking beyond the biomedical model. The authors incorporate a broad range of effective teaching methods in their chapters. Even more importantly, the book does not shy away from uncomfortable discussions, challenging us all to think beyond the colonial lens through which the health and psychology fields have historically operated."
—Dr. Mary Cwik, *Center for American Indian Health, Johns Hopkins School of Public Health, USA*

"This is a landmark publication. The lack of cultural safety is one of our biggest challenges in the US health care system. We need to centralize the experience of diverse voices and communities, especially the hidden/marginalized, if we are to achieve health equity. Cultural safety is the most comprehensive approach to cultural discourse in health care. Training a workforce that has the ability work safely with cultural difference and to address the persistent inequities in the history and system of health and health care should be our #1 priority. I dream that someday we can require cultural safety throughout our health care system. This book provides the necessary introduction to cultural safety for health care in the United States."

—Prof. Nathaniel Mohatt, *School of Medicine, University of Colorado, USA*

Contents

1	**Introduction and Terminology**	1
	Chapter Objectives	2
	Overview	2
	Cultural Safety: Some Key Concepts	6
	How We Talk About This Topic: Terminology and Definitions	9
	Race and Ethnicity	12
	Informal Terminology	16
	Colonization–Relevance for Health and Human Services Practice	19
	Decolonizing Practice	21
	Conclusion	22
	References	23
2	**Culture-Focused Frameworks for Service Delivery**	25
	Chapter Objectives	26
	Culture and Health	26
	Trans-cultural or Multicultural Practice	27
	Cultural Safety	29

	Other Cultural Frameworks	30
	Cultural Awareness	31
	Cultural Sensitivity	31
	Cultural Competence	31
	Cultural Humility	35
	Cultural Responsiveness	36
	Summary of Concepts	36
	Conclusion	41
	References	42
3	**Cultural Safety**	45
	Chapter Objectives	45
	What Is Cultural Safety and What It Is Not	46
	Pathways to Cultural Safety	46
	Cultural Safety Principles	57
	Conclusion	62
	References	63
4	**Models of Health and Well-Being**	65
	Chapter Objectives	65
	Definitions of Health	66
	Models of Health	69
	Social Determinants of Health	73
	The Principles of Primary Health Care	77
	Health Beliefs and Models of Care	84
	Conclusion	87
	References	87
5	**History Taking**	89
	Chapter Objectives	89
	History and Health	90
	Relevance of History	91
	Colonization and the Impact on Health Today	96
	Past Policies	100
	Key Dates and Events in History	101
	Government Responses	102
	Definitions of Identity	102

	Current Policy	105
	Policy and Cultural Safety	107
	Case Study: Native American Boarding Schools	108
	Conclusion	111
	References	111
6	**Consuming Research**	113
	Chapter Objectives	113
	What Is Research?	114
	Diunital Versus Dichotomous Logic and Worldviews	116
	Assessing Information	119
	Research Methods	122
	Randomized Controlled Trials	122
	Ethics and Research	124
	Community-Based Participatory Research	126
	Special Topic: Culture and Population Migration: Female Circumcision	127
	Conclusion	133
	References	133
7	**Determinants of Health**	137
	Chapter Objectives	137
	Determinants of Health Explained	138
	Culture and Identity as Determinants of Health and Well-Being	141
	Education	142
	Employment and Wealth	144
	Housing, Overcrowding, and Houselessness	146
	Racism and Discrimination	148
	Cultural Safety and Racism and Discrimination	154
	Conclusion	162
	References	163
8	**Stats and Maps**	165
	Chapter Objectives	165
	Awareness	166
	Epidemiology and COVID-19	166

	Life Expectancy	168
	Demographic Profile	171
	Urban, Suburban, Rural	174
	Age Distributions	177
	Maps	180
	Critical Thinking About the Statistics: Identity	184
	Revisiting Identity, Languages	186
	Conclusion	188
	References	189
9	**Special Interest and Priority Areas**	**191**
	Chapter Objectives	191
	What Are Our Priorities?	192
	Healthy People: U.S. Priorities	193
	Chronic Diseases	197
	Infectious and Parasitic Diseases	200
	Infant and Maternal Health	202
	Risky and High-Risk Substance Use	203
	Opioid Epidemic in the U.S.	205
	Mental Health and Social and Emotional Well-Being	206
	Aging	209
	Assessments	210
	(Dis)abilities	211
	Conclusion	215
	References	215
10	**Capacity and Resilience**	**217**
	Chapter Objectives	217
	Concepts: Capacity, Resilience, Cultural Vitality	218
	Role of Health and Human Services Professionals	224
	Changing the Discourse	227
	Forgiveness and Reconciliation	229
	Traditional Knowledges	230
	Success Stories	234
	Black Lives Matter	236
	Conclusion	237
	References	237

11 Intercultural Communication — 239
- Chapter Objectives — 239
- Intercultural or Cross-Cultural Interactions — 240
- Communication in Health and Human Services — 240
- The Influence of Accents on Communications — 242
- Limited English Proficiency (LEP) — 245
- Working with Interpreters — 253
- Health Literacy — 254
- Conclusion — 259
- References — 259

12 Comparable Contexts — 261
- Chapter Objectives — 262
- Indigenous Peoples in a Comparable Global Context — 262
- Colonization in Australia, the U.S., Canada, and Aotearoa/New Zealand — 264
- Canada — 265
- The United States — 266
- Aotearoa/ New Zealand — 270
- Australia — 271
- Some Comparisons — 273
- 'How Indigenous Are You?' — 275
- Terminology — 276
- Disease and Colonization — 278
- The Most Recent Contacts — 279
- Population and Health Status of Indigenous Peoples in a Global context — 280
- Can We Fix Our Problems by Doing What Others Do? — 280
- Decolonization and Health and Human Service Professionals — 281
- Conclusion — 283
- References — 284

13 Reflection as a Tool of Culturally Safe Practice — 287
- Chapter Objectives — 288
- Reflection — 288
- What Is Reflective Practice? — 289

Cultural Safety Principles for Practice: An Opportunity
to Reflect 294
Practice Strategies 300
Cultural Safety of Health and Human Service
Professionals 303
Conclusion 304
References 304

Index 307

List of Figures

Fig. 1.1	Equal treatment does not provide equal outcomes (*Image Credit* #the4thbox Equality/Equity/Liberation image collaboration between Center for Story-based Strategy & Interactive Institute for Social Change)	3
Fig. 3.1	Original stages of cultural safety as defined by Ramsden (Taylor & Thompson-Guerin, 2019)	47
Fig. 3.2	An aspirational model of cultural safety—always incorporating new understandings and reflections to enhance culturally safe care, as defined by recipients (Taylor & Thompson-Guerin, 2019)	49
Fig. 5.1	Indigenous and European occupation of *Great Turtle Island*, now called the U.S.	92
Fig. 7.1	Impact of educational disadvantage (Taylor & Thompson-Guerin, 2019)	143
Fig. 7.2	A visual of the differences between equality, equity, reality and liberation (Image credit: #the4thbox Equality/Equity/Liberation image collaboration between *Center for Story-based Strategy* and *Interactive Institute for Social Change*. Reality panel created by Andrew Weizeman)	153

Fig. 7.3	Chevara Orrin	160
Fig. 8.1	Life expectancy for male and female and White, Black, and Hispanic (*Source* Arias, 2016)	170
Fig. 8.2	Population pyramids for Native Hawaiian and Pacific Islanders (NHPI), Asian, AI/AN, Black and White males and females in the U.S.	179

List of Tables

Table 2.1	Cultural frameworks, some strengths, and limitations	38
Table 4.1	Key differences between biomedical and social approaches to health	71
Table 6.1	A comparison of diunital and dichotomous logic or worldview with examples	117
Table 8.1	American Indian and Alaska Native population (alone or in combination) by state and (% of total 2010 state population)	173
Table 8.2	Geographic distribution of healthcare professionals, 2010 (%)	176
Table 8.3	Median age by sex and race in the U.S	177
Table 9.1	*Healthy People 2020* leading health indicators and objectives	195
Table 11.1	Elements of healthcare communications in the U.S	246
Table 12.1	Comparison of Indigenous populations and treaty status in four countries	267
Table 13.1	Layers of reflection (adapted from Johns, 2017)	290

1

Introduction and Terminology

Culture is all pervading in our lives—especially when we view culture as more than ethnicity or race. However, when we are embedded within and surrounded by others of our own culture, our cultural identity is often experienced in a less conscious way. For some people, until they encounter cultural difference or dissonance, their own culture may barely come into consciousness. Raising consciousness about the role of culture in health psychology and health and human services work is a critical step in providing care and service that is not only competent, but culturally safe for all.

In this chapter, we introduce the main ideas of this book—cultural safety as a preferred way of working as professionals, the need to decolonize our professional practice, and the importance of using informed terminology when working in a range of cultural contexts.

Chapter Objectives

After completing this chapter, you should be able to:

- define cultural safety in relation to health psychology and health and human services
- identify appropriate terminology and rationales for their use
- examine the relevance of colonization to your own practice or professional aspiration
- identify strategies to decolonize your practice

Overview

In this book, *A Cultural Safety Approach to Health Psychology*, we apply the concept of cultural safety to the field of health psychology and professional work in the health and human services in the U.S. 'Cultural' differences are most often thought about as those more overt differences related to race or ethnicity—language, foods, modes of dress, rituals, and behaviors. However, cultural safety as both a philosophy and model of practice, looks at culture as also including differences in terms of age, sexualities, genders, religion, migration status, abilities, or socioeconomic background. Where professionals and their clients differ in these areas, evidence shows this can be a major factor in contributing to health disparities.

Many books continue to buy into narrow 'biomedical' and 'biopsychosocial' frameworks that perpetuate individualistic, capitalistic, and medicalized viewpoints. In this book, we explore cultural safety as both a philosophy and way of working within a social model of health as an alternative approach to understanding health and illness. Furthermore, as health and illness can be directly and indirectly linked to our and other countries' colonizing pasts, we apply a decolonizing framework to professional practice.

So, we are barely into the first chapter and we have already talked about culture as a major determinant of health—culture in its broadest sense—and the impact of our colonial past on health and social care.

Educating health and human service professionals is an incredibly important, as well as daunting, task in a current climate that is often ambivalent at the least and hostile at the worst. In some sectors, the teaching of cultural diversity, difference, or acknowledgment of the impact of cultural dissonance has been seen as 'dangerous' ideas by those who seek to deny that there is any problem with the way healthcare and human services are provided. After all, we treat everyone the same, don't we? Even if that could be accepted as true, equal treatment, as we will hope to show, does not always translate to equal outcomes. Treating everyone the same, can in fact, aggravate existing disparities, by assuming everyone exists on a level playing field (Fig. 1.1).

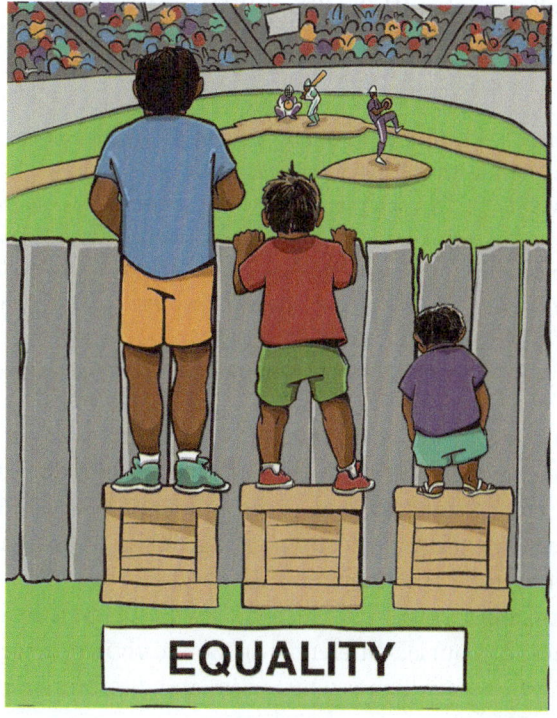

Fig. 1.1 Equal treatment does not provide equal outcomes (*Image Credit* #the4thbox Equality/Equity/Liberationimage collaboration between Center for Story-based Strategy & Interactive Institute for Social Change)

This above picture shows that while treating everyone the same seems appropriate, failing to take into account individual differences (in this case, physical differences, rather than cultural), can prove ineffective in providing appropriate support. What if the difference in accessing care or services was economic background, race or ethnicity, sexuality, religion, or gender? It would be easy to see this as discriminatory and yet it sounds reasonable in theory, to treat everyone 'equally.'

There is a myriad of examples that could be cited, of cultural differences negatively affecting the health and well-being of individuals and groups. Research has long shown that differences in cultural background between clients and professionals can lead to poorer outcomes, shorter consultations, lower quality information exchange, and more (Bailey et al., 2017; Ben et al., 2017; Tello, 2017).

> **Reading**
> A recent article identified physician–patient racial differences as implicated in higher deaths of newborn Black babies.
> Greenwood, B. N., Hardeman, R. R., Huang, L., & Sojourner, A. (2020). Physician–patient racial concordance and disparities in birthing mortality for newborns. *Proceedings of the National Academy of Sciences, 117*(35), 21194–21200, https://doi.org/10.1073/pnas.1913405117.

This is not suggesting any conscious or deliberate act on the part of physicians to provide poorer standards of care. What it does demonstrate are the very real cultural biases that can influence how care is provided, such as a lack of adequate history taking, assumptions, stereotyping, discrimination, and 'othering' (i.e., the tendency to view the other as exotic and usually lesser), that can occur without even being aware of it. Sometimes, of course, differences in how care is provided may well occur with awareness, which is why racism and discrimination awareness are also necessary features of cultural safety.

Much of the literature on disparities and cultural differences, as above, has focused on culture as it relates to race or ethnicity only. To date, the emphases in healthcare and human services and policy settings have largely expected vulnerable and marginalized people—usually those perceived to be 'the other'—to change themselves in order to change their outcomes. Less attention has been given to the changes that members of the majority or dominant groups and systems could and should make to provide more effective, or safe, care, and environments.

Here it's important to say that language and terminology will be mentioned a lot—because language matters. The words we choose are usually through a specific cultural lens and are often laden or contested. In health care, the system in and of itself, as well as the providers within that system, are 'dominant', or hold power, over those in their care in terms of access to particular knowledge or resources. But we do not mean dominant in any value sense or in the sense of any inherent quality. When we use the word 'minority', we do not mean 'less than' in any judgment of value, but in the sense of being 'outnumbered' or unequal in power relationships or access to particular resources or knowledges within a specific situation.

A recent quote from Janel Cubbage emphasizes the importance of reflecting on what specific language actually means: 'We are not minorities, we have been minoritized. We are not underrepresented. We have been systematically excluded. Language matters' (15 November, 2020, Twitter @janel cubbage).

So, in healthcare and human services, whatever the difference between professionals and clients, rather than expecting clients to 'fit in', cultural safety asks those in the 'dominant' role to examine their professional practice to accommodate client needs, where possible. There will be times where such changes are not possible, but cultural safety is about *how* things are done, as much as *what* is done. If you cannot provide a female staff member for someone who would prefer this, for example, the way this is navigated moving forward will determine the cultural safety of the encounter. Sometimes even a brief acknowledgment that you would like to be able to offer the choice, but staffing or situations at the time prevent this, is enough for someone to feel 'safer'.

Poor health and conditions in the U.S. are the result of a multiplicity of circumstances, histories, attitudes, and beliefs and therefore need to be thought about within this multiplicity of contexts. No one wants to get diabetes, for example. Biomedical explanations can only go so far in understanding and addressing such a health issue. Diet and sedentary lifestyles may explain part of the cause, but what explains the inequitable access to fresh and affordable foods? Eating healthy is not simply a matter of 'choice'. How are we to understand and intervene for more active lifestyles when not all neighborhoods are safe?

If we, as a nation, could figure out how to improve health, wellbeing, and living conditions for those among us who are most at need, who are most vulnerable and marginalized in terms of health, and for everyone who seeks care, what might be the implications for health and U.S. society as a whole? At an individual level, if we learned how to deliver services so that outcomes mattered, this could improve health for everyone. Organizationally, if we learned how to structure our systems so that no one was left behind, that everyone benefitted, we would have an organizational structure coveted by all. And if our policies were such that everyone mattered, in real ways, and that policies did not present barriers but facilitated culturally safe care, again, *everyone* would benefit. This would mean providing care and services that are not delivered *regardless* of cultural differences, but *regardful of* and able to accommodate differences. Apart from all the mutual benefit, health is a universal human right and whenever there is disparity within our nation, we are all diminished. We can and must do better.

Cultural Safety: Some Key Concepts

Cultural safety, as both a philosophy and a model for practice, was developed by Māori (the Indigenous people of New Zealand) midwives in New Zealand. It is the preferred model for educating health professionals in New Zealand, Australia, and Canada but has been slower to catch on in the U.S. or to be applied in the social and human services or psychology domains. We hope that by the end of this book, we will have demonstrated the strong relevance this concept has for the U.S. and how an Indigenous-derived approach can be transformative for all.

Cultural safety is defined by the New Zealand Nursing Council of New Zealand (2011, p. 4) as:

The effective nursing practice of a person or family from another culture, and is determined by that person or family. Culture includes, but is not restricted to, age or generation; gender; sexual orientation; occupation and socioeconomic status; ethnic origin or migrant experience; religious or spiritual belief; and disability.

The nurse delivering the nursing service will have undertaken a process of reflection on his or her own cultural identity and will recognize the impact that his or her personal culture has on his or her professional practice. Unsafe cultural practice comprises any action, which diminishes, demeans or disempowers the cultural identity and well-being of an individual.

Look at the key terms in the above definition: effective care; determined by the (recipient of care); cultural difference broadly defined; reflection on practice; and the professional recognizing the impact of their own culture on their professional practice. The onus for any adaptation in the care relationship is firmly on the professional—a way of mitigating potential power imbalances for the client or patient.

Cultural competence, the model more commonly used in the U.S., has been defined as the knowledge, awareness, and skills aimed at providing services that promotes and advances cultural diversity and recognizes the uniqueness of self and others in communities (American Psychological Association, 2017). Simply, cultural safety is distinguished from cultural competence in that culturally safe practice is determined by the recipient of care and this is made explicit, while in cultural competence it is not made explicit—though one might assume that 'knowledge, awareness and skills' are assessed by supervisors or others in charge. Both cultural safety and cultural competence require self-reflection, but cultural competence emphasizes the knowledge base of the professional. This knowledge base often relates to specific cultural practices that can be perceived as fixed and able to be categorized, whereby, cultural safety focuses more on the diversity both within and between 'cultural' groups and the dynamics of cultural interactions. We explore these differences more in later chapters.

Cultural safety is also one approach that recognizes that health and well-being today is linked to our colonizing histories and asks health professionals to 'decolonize' their practice. There may be some readers who are unclear about how history influences health care and human services today. However, understanding that colonization is a process of asserting power and dominance, then we can begin to understand that power relationships in health care and human services require attention. A decolonizing approach is woven throughout the book, offering ways that professionals might examine their own practice and work to ensure more equitable power relationships with clients.

The U.S. was brought into existence through the dispossession of land from the Indigenous inhabitants and then built and exploited using people who were stolen from their homelands. These remarks are not said to elicit guilt or anger—they are a matter of historical fact and part of the 'history-taking' that any good health or human service professional should conduct to inform their practice. The impact of colonization on health and well-being is critical to our understanding and provision of care and services today. But as the question arose earlier, shouldn't our services and care be the same, no matter who we are working with? The U.S., as a multicultural society, should include everyone, right? Why focus on particular groups?

> **Scenario**
> During a conversation at a family gathering, the conversation turned to health care. A father stated that he didn't believe his taxes or payment for health insurance should go toward paying for people who didn't have their own health insurance or for things such as women's health which did not directly benefit him. He had always taken responsibility for his own health, worked hard, and looked after himself and his family.
> - How would you respond to these comments? Do they align with your own view closely, somewhat or not at all? Give a rationale for your answer. (Please note, a rationale is a reasoned case, **not** an opinion.)
> - What worldview is reflected in this approach to health?
> - A few months later, the father ended up unemployed due to a business closure that meant the loss of his health insurance. Not long after, his wife was diagnosed with breast cancer.
> - Do these developments change any of your responses above?

> "We are only as strong as the most vulnerable person in our community, so now more than ever it is imperative for us to decolonize from individualism and reconnect with ways of community care" (Begay, 2020). What is important to acknowledge is that any one of us can be made 'vulnerable' by circumstances often beyond our control.

How We Talk About This Topic: Terminology and Definitions

To begin this and any conversation regarding culture, we need to find out what words to use to describe groups and people before we explore other topics. Establishing the correct terminology to use is like making an introduction and telling someone your name—specifically how you want to be addressed, which itself may depend on the cultural context in which it is used. Already, we are using the term 'client' to describe those receiving services or care. We could have also used terms such as 'patient' or 'service user' or many other terms (see McLaughlin, 2009). These terms come in and out of fashion and can be preferred or opposed depending on location, the group you are working with, and many other variables. While 'client' isn't a perfect term because of the inherent power implication in its use, in the absence of more appropriate term, it is the term we have chosen to use. As with other terms and labels, seek to understand the preferred terms with your clients and workplace.

We will be discussing a range of identities including gender, race, ethnicity, sexualities, abilities, religions, age, and socioeconomic status. The range of cultures and identities discussed in this book are inherently diverse and anything but static. Therefore, we need to set some parameters for the use of terminology from this point.

Acronyms and abbreviations are sometimes used for brevity and identification, such as LGBTQIAP+ and many variations of this abbreviation. However, there is quite a bit of discussion and debate about the use of abbreviations (also called initialism) because they have the potential to exclude some or assume all individuals and groups are happy to be identified together under such labels. Here, these letters can stand for Lesbian, Gay, Bisexual, Transgender or Transsexual or Trans* as an inclusive term, Queer, or GenderQueer, or Questioning, Intersex, Asexual or Ally, and Pansexual. A ' + ' at the end is a way to include anyone else who doesn't fit into any of the other categories. There is not universal acceptance even within groups for whom these terms apply. Overall, these initials or this abbreviation are about sexualities and gender identities. Keep in mind that sexuality is different from gender identity, but these are often categorized together. A more recently suggested acronym is SAGA, for sexuality and gender acceptance. Acronyms can also be used in medical or government writings (such as AI/AN for American Indian/Alaska Native) and may partly result from publishing requirements to shorten any phrases frequently used so as to reduce costs. While some people and groups may be perfectly fine with various abbreviations or acronyms, others may not. Abbreviations and acronyms can be offensive to some people. Think about the impact of reducing to an acronym or abbreviation or a plus sign something that is an important description of your identity.

These examples highlight the need to always check with people what their preferred identifiers or descriptors are as an inherent part of a cultural safety approach. Use of various abbreviations, acronyms, or other descriptors can change depending on the person, their age, the geographic region you are in, or many other factors such as academic conventions versus common use. The need to check current and local usage is a key message of this book, as shown in each chapter section called "Making It Local."

> **Scenario**
> A new client has come to the mental health clinic. The receptionist asks them their name and the person responds: 'Amy'. When Amy provides the receptionist with their health insurance card, the receptionist says, 'This card says 'David' and David is a male name; what is your name?' Amy responds that the card has her legal name, but she prefers to be called Amy and her pronouns are she/her. The receptionist says, 'So are

you a male or a female'? And proceeds to refer to Amy in all future correspondence as 'he' and 'him'.
- How might the receptionist have handled this engagement more sensitively?
- What assumptions has the receptionist made about gender identities and legal names?
- How might this interaction impact on Amy's healthcare seeking in the future?

When the receptionist has realized that Amy is transgender, she says to Amy, "Oh I don't care about any of that, 'to each his own'; everyone can live their own life the way they want!".

- Does this statement make the situation more or less acceptable?
- What might the impact be on Amy to always have to explain her identity?

Simply starting a conversation about this topic may seem fraught with difficulty. Some might think that the potential to offend is overwhelming and there is too much 'political correctness'. Readers might therefore opt to avoid discussions relating to cultures and identities. But why do we emphasize the importance of trying to use correct terminology? Is it 'political correctness' and what does that actually mean? Could it be that when something is deemed an example of 'political correctness' it is more likely to be a resistance to acknowledging that some language, attitudes, and behaviors marginalize and demean others? It is easy to make mistakes especially in interactions with people for whom you have little experience or knowledge but, as we will discuss more in future chapters, learning through reflective practice means acknowledging any mistakes and re-orienting your approach. Indeed, it may well be that by the time this book is being read, some of our own language, terminology, and definitions may well be outdated or unacceptable.

Race and Ethnicity

Race and ethnicity are terms that are often used interchangeably, but there are important differences between the concepts that warrant discussion. Race is a concept that usually assumes biological or genetic differences between groups of people. It is often determined by differences in skin color and facial or other physical characteristics. This way of thinking was prominent in the early nineteenth century with scientists such as Samuel George Morton from Philadelphia, who believed that there were multiple racial creations. He studied this theory by exploring skull differences of people from all around the world, ultimately determining that Europeans had the highest brain capacity (and therefore intelligence), and Africans and Aboriginal Australians had the smallest. It is not a surprising result that a European researcher found Europeans to be superior. We talk about this kind of bias more in the Research chapter. This work was later used to 'justify' enslaving certain people and other racist treatment. This obsession with collecting skulls for 'scientific' research caused considerable distress and continues to cause distress to those whose family member's remains were removed without regard for the impact of such acts.

> **Reading**
> See this article about decolonizing museums:
> Hunt, T. (2019, June 29). Should museums return their colonial artefacts? *The Guardian*. https://www.theguardian.com/culture/2019/jun/29/should-museums-return-their-colonial-artefacts.

Morton's research, and that of others similar to his, is now considered to be 'scientific racism' because of how racism was legitimized through 'scientific' methods. When defined in this way, it is a highly problematic concept because presumed biological or genetic differences between large groups of people do not exist (Goldberg, 1990). The often-cited information here is that there are genetically more differences *within* groups of people than there are *between* them. This means that there are no definitive genes or clusters of genes or biological markers that determine whether someone is White or Black, for example. However, the use of 'race' as a term to categorize people is perpetuated by, for example, the use of these categories in almost all documentation in the U.S. (such as on census forms or medical documents), which has incredible power internationally in influencing ideas.

Considering 'race' as a biological or genetic reality does not have a basis in science and has led to many problems. Sociologists, psychologists, anthropologists, and other social scientists conceptualize 'race' as a *social construction*, with political, social, and economic meanings with a long history. Even if we know that race is not a biological reality, race, as a social construction, has consequences, which are certainly real. However, it can be difficult to know how the term '*race*' is being used—is it being used to infer only biological differences, or is it being used within the broader, socially constructed, concept? In the U.S., according to the Office of Management and Budget (OMB), the concept of 'race' is used when referring to White, Black or African American, Asian, Native Hawaiian or Other Pacific Islander and American Indian or Alaska Native, but 'ethnicity' is the term used when referring to people who identify as Hispanic or Latino (OMB, 1997). People who identify as Hispanic or Latino can be Cuban, Mexican, Puerto Rican, South or Central American, or other Spanish culture. For the 2020 U.S. Census, people could identify their 'origin' as Hispanic, Spanish or Latino and could 'be of any race' (Marks & Jones, 2020).

Resources

For more details on language use relating to the terms Hispanic, Latino, and more, see this History article: Simon, Y. (2020). Latino, Hispanic, Latinx, Chicano: The history behind the terms. History.com https://www.history.com/news/hispanic-latino-latinx-chicano-background.

With a warning that some people may find the content distressing, watch the YouTube clip 'The Morton Collection of Human Skulls: Full interview at Penn' at: https://www.youtube.com/watch?v=mMVzPCOut1w.

In the U.S. Census, people are also asked to indicate their place of birth, their citizenship, and year of entry (U.S. Census Bureau, n.d.). Race and ethnicity in the U.S. Census are based on self-identification, although the American Indian or Alaska Native question asks respondents to indicate their 'enrolled or principal tribe(s)'. *Ethnicity* in common usage is defined as an identity that is based on shared cultural values or practices.

Think about what it would be like for you as an individual to be referred to by an imposed label. We will repeatedly remind readers to find out what is preferred locally from credible sources—ask people of the relevant group for the accepted terminology for any given region, age group, or person—rather than make assumptions. Look at the various terminology that might be used to describe Native Americans, American Indians, or the Indigenous Peoples of the U.S. Throughout the U.S. there will be differences in what terms are accepted and even what terms might be offensive to some. We have used the term 'Indigenous' at times throughout the book for readability and brevity with no disrespect intended or we have used the terminology employed in the sources we are citing, such as the U.S. Census Bureau, which uses 'American Indian and Alaska Native' in most publications. Where we refer to specific populations we have tried to ensure that the accepted identifiers have been used.

Before the colonization of the U.S., the terminologies 'Native American' or 'American Indian' did not exist as a form of self-identification for the peoples who lived in this country. These labels or identifiers were imposed by the colonizing groups. Even today, many people identify by their tribal group, but some do use these other terms. It is important to be aware that there may be multiple spellings for different language groupings, tribes, and community names.

Look at the label 'American' for example. Americans are quite a diverse group, with around 330 million people in the U.S. alone, clearly all 'Americans' are not the same. But then what about Central Americans or South Americans? Are they, too, 'Americans'? Do all 'Americans' have flags flying on their front porches and are they all largely unaware about the rest of the world and only able to speak English? Using these examples, you might see how terminology can be problematic.

In this book we have ensured the capitalization of 'Indigenous' when referring specifically to Indigenous Peoples of the U.S. According to the conventions of the American Psychological Association, we also capitalize all racial or ethnic descriptors, such as Black or White or Asian or Hispanic. Descriptors such as African American or Asian American are generally only used when referring to sources that have used those descriptors such as the U.S. Census Bureau. Not all Black people who live in the U.S. are 'from' Africa or were born in or consider themselves 'American'. While some might see using the term 'Black' as being offensive, for many, it has been adopted as a signifier of a culture and identity. The term 'African American' is generally used to indicate the history of African origin for people who embrace the 'American' identity, but again, these labels and their use can be complicated, and one should not make assumptions about their use.

Overall, people vary in their preferences for different descriptors, and, as we will learn with culturally safe practice, it is always important to ask people what their preferences are. This is not just a matter of being pedantic or politically correct but rather it is a matter of showing the same respect you would expect for yourself. As with the other terminology we discussed, it is important to understand that at least for some people, it can be highly offensive, and even considered racist, when these terms are not capitalized. Would you write your own name or nationality with small case? Probably not, but the writer, professor, and feminist, bell hooks, intentionally does not capitalize her name as a way to subvert common conventions. To capitalize her name would be disrespectful. As professionals, it is our responsibility to be aware of these possibilities and to do our best to not 'diminish, disempower, or demean' someone's cultural identity, which includes the terminology we use to describe people.

> **Reading**
> For a helpful insight into the use and misuse of the acronym POC, for People of Color, see Copes, C. (2021). Can y'all please learn how to

> use "POC"? on Medium.com. https://medium.com/an-injustice/can-y-all-please-learn-how-to-use-poc-f9931a31bcbc.

As may be already apparent, there is a diversity of terminology and respectful ways of talking with and about groups of people. Many organizations have style guides regarding terminology, and you are encouraged to seek these out at the local level.

> **Critical Thinking**
> - What is your response to the issue of terminology? Do you think it really matters or is this merely political correctness? Why do you think some requests for change are labeled as political correctness? Who benefits when something is labeled as political correctness?
> - Think of an example where you have been referred to by a label imposed by someone else. How did you feel about it?
> - What cultural groups are in your region—remember culture is more than ethnicity? How do they identify themselves?
> - It is essential that every effort be made to find out and use the *locally* and *culturally* appropriate terminology in your discussions. How might you find out this information? Where would you look? Who would you ask?

Informal Terminology

Many people frequently use informal terms to refer to themselves and others in daily life. Usage of these terms can vary regionally and between groups of people, and what is affectionate or acceptable in some areas or by some people could be offensive in others. Perhaps the most contentious racial slur in the U.S. is the 'N' word. Though it can be heard in music, movies, comedy, and between individuals, it is one of the most-taboo words to be used today. Indeed, even in this book, we write the 'N' word without actually writing it, because, to do so, might well be seen by many as racist (McWhorter, 2019).

The use of certain terms can be an act of reclamation of power—a way of taking the intended offense and hurt away. This is not an invitation to use such terminology. It is not our place to give such permission. You may have heard certain groups using what are usually considered derogatory names within their own peer group and it would be easy to believe this was inviting the same kind of informality, only to find the recipients have taken offense.

How will you know what names are appropriate to use? Ask! Ask the person how they want to be addressed and do the same in return. Don't assume because you have heard others using a nickname or other informal term to refer to someone, that it is OK for you to do the same. We asked above, and ask again, can you think of a time when you have been addressed in a way that was offensive to you? For some young people, being called 'son', 'boy', or 'young lady' for example, could feel demeaning.

Activity
- For this activity, you will need to form a small group, perhaps with others studying this book or maybe with your family or other people you live with. Each member of the group should explain to their group one way in which they identify themselves and why. This could be their identity linked to their gender, their profession, home state or city, marital status, or all of these. Before you get started, your group should establish some rules. They might include, for example, respecting others and their choice not to identify personal information about themselves. Individual anonymity should be maintained both inside and outside the group.
- An alternative to verbally introducing yourselves, ask everyone to depict their identity/identities in a drawing. Art can be a wonderful activity that pushes people outside of their 'cultural norm' or comfort zone.
- How did people identify themselves? Reflect on the reasons people gave as to why their identity was important. Some of the common self-applied labels include marital status, parenting roles, religion, interests, employment background, and ethnic heritage or racial identity. Did

anyone identify themselves by their cultural, racial, or ethnic background? For example, if someone identified themselves as 'half Irish', 'half Black', 'one quarter Filipino' or 'Colombian', ask how they might feel if the government used that classification to restrict their travel, places of residence, rights, etc. Think about how a term such as 'half-blood' can be offensive and may cause harm when the origin and intent are not understood. Similarly, are there terms that have been assumed to be offensive that are embraced? Who decides what terms are acceptable or not?

- If you cannot do the activity in a group, recall the last time you were in a social situation with people you were not familiar with. How did people introduce themselves? What was the context of the social situation, and did that influence how people introduced themselves? For example, if you are at a work get-together, people introduce themselves through their job title ('I'm the manager'), but if you are in a family situation, people may introduce themselves through family connections ('I'm Stella's husband').

Scenario

A mother with two adolescent children has come to the emergency department with one of the children having possibly broken their arm skateboarding. The mother completes the forms and has ticked the box 'Black'. The nurse looked at the form and begins entering the data into the system. Based on the mother's appearance, the nurse suggests that perhaps she has made a mistake on the form—that she has wrongly ticked 'Black'.

Critical Thinking

- What assumptions has the nurse made about identity?
- What impact might this have on this family's experience of health care?
- How might this impact on this mother's experience of the system?
- How likely is she to feel welcome there and come back again?
- What message do the children get about their identities?

Through critical reflection (discussed more in Chapter 13), health and human service professionals and students can develop readily transferable skills to the care of any individual or group. You will likely work with people who have experienced a variety of influences on their health and well-being, such as loss, trauma, resilience, survival, grief, pride, capacity, health, and illness. Challenging your own assumptions, stereotypes, and possible biases is an important principle of culturally safe practice.

Making It Local
- What relevance does learning about culture and cultural safety have for your own professional practice or intended practice? Write down your expectations now so that you will have them to review when you reach the end of this book.
- What do you know about the local population groups and people in your region or specific location? Please ensure you investigate your assertion thoroughly.

Colonization–Relevance for Health and Human Services Practice

We have mentioned colonization as relevant to health and human services practice, but how many agree with this idea? Colonization or colonialism is a construct that sounds as if it belongs in the history books, rather than a book for health and human services professionals. However, colonization is not a relic of the past and post-colonialism does not imply something that is over. It can also simply mean 'the period since'. Colonizing practices continue today. Colonization is about dominance and asserting power over and exploiting one's own privilege. It's about accepting systematic and institutionalized biases that disadvantage some and benefit others. The healthcare and human services industries in the U.S. are certainly dominated by the biomedical or Western construct of medicine and health care. As a wealthy, powerful country, the U.S.

healthcare system focuses largely on treatments and pharmacotherapeutics with environmental and social determinants of health remaining under-resourced and undervalued.

Look at the lack of readiness faced by the healthcare system in dealing with the COVID-19 pandemic and the value placed on a vaccine rather than low-cost strategies like social distancing, stringent handwashing, and masks in public. Indeed, with so much money going toward vaccinations and other mitigation strategies, would that money be better spent on health promotion and prevention of illnesses or pre-existing conditions? With the knowledge that people with 'pre-existing conditions' are most at risk, shouldn't we focus on reducing the causes of 'pre-existing conditions' such as improved housing, reduced pollution, increased access to healthy foods, safer living environments, and better working conditions? Of course, once a pandemic has struck, the priorities shift to deal with the immediate risks, leading to a vicious cycle of action in some areas and inaction in others. However, decisions about our health should not be either/or, as we will discuss in the chapter on Models of Health. Health care in this time, perhaps more overtly than in other times, has been politicized and, in a sense, colonized, exposing and aggravating existing disparities even further.

Colonization as an historic event, however, can also be directly implicated in health outcomes of various populations today. Most of the groups affected by colonial pasts are the Indigenous, Black and Hispanic peoples, who, as a result of history, were dispossessed, dispersed from their homelands, and decimated through conflict, disease, or other causes. There is considerable evidence that the detrimental effects of colonization have influenced health outcomes through successive generations, in areas such as mental health and chronic diseases, maternal and child health, substance misuse, and more. One example of how colonization has affected health today is the radical change from an Indigenous diet to a Western diet, which has contributed to whole families being susceptible to diabetes, heart and kidney disease.

Without an understanding of our colonizing pasts, including policies and practices that have led to a mistrust and fear of some health and other services, cultural safety will be less attainable. Colonizing practices are fairly universal—dominate, assert power over, force people to comply, divide and conquer, suppress cultures and languages, restrict and remove freedoms, and control information and knowledge. Colonization doesn't have to involve armies engaged in conflict. Think about the language still used in health care when someone chooses to leave the hospital without completing treatment—they are noted as 'absconding', 'discharged against medical advice', or 'non-compliant'. These labels perpetuate or maintain colonization of our professional practices by implying the person is guilty of some wrongdoing rather than acting with agency and making different choices.

Decolonizing Practice

What then does it mean to decolonize healthcare and human services practice? From a cultural safety standpoint, it means making sure that we do not assert power over or dominate those of a different cultural background to ourselves. Ultimately, as professionals providing services, we automatically are in a position of power over those in our care. Clients come to us because they believe we can help or that we have something they need. But how can we reduce this power differential and be more mindful of how it might impact our services and outcomes? As a start, we examine our own biases and stereotyped ideas and assumptions, and we engage in dialogue with the clients to provide care that they will deem culturally safe. So many interactions in health and human services can be made culturally safe by adherence to these few simple principles. As cultural safety is an ongoing aspiration, there is opportunity for reflection and improvement in the ways of working.

> **Scenario**
> A young boy in the pediatric department asked for a toy from the toy box using his first language, Spanish. The large male nurse loudly stated that he would not give the boy any toys while he was speaking 'a foreign language'. 'No, when you stop talking in that language and ask me properly in English, then I'll give it to you'.

> - What lessons did the child learn about the world in this one small exchange?
> - What underlying message does the young boy get about his own language and identity?
> - What did he learn about power?
> - What colonizing strategy is evident in the nurse's response?
> - How might this scene be made more culturally safe for all participants?
> - Who is in the best position to change practice?

Conclusion

In this chapter, we discussed relevant terminology and asked the reader to investigate locally appropriate terminologies. We also sought to examine the relevance of identities to individual practice. We discussed rationales for studying the impacts of colonization on health and outlined some strategies for decolonizing practice.

Some key cultural safety principles have already emerged:

- Simply ask how someone wants to be addressed; respect how they choose to identify without questioning, assuming, or stereotyping.
- Consider the influence of history and decolonize practice by not continuing to impose and disempower individuals or make assumptions.
- Reflect on your use of language and terminology. Identify the origins of terminology and acceptability in the local context.
- Think about who has power when different terminology is used or when it is assumed, and who makes the assumptions.

These principles are applicable to working with anyone of a different cultural background to yourself. One assumption that is probably safe to make is that, as a professional providing services, everyone you are working with is different to you. Culture can be generational, social, religious, or any difference that exists between you and the client or recipient of care. The following chapters will present an argument for the use of cultural safety as an underlying philosophical approach to health and human services.

References

American Psychological Association. (2017). *Multicultural guidelines: An ecological approach to context, identity, and intersectionality*. Retrieved January 25, 2021 from: http://www.apa.org/about/policy/multicultural-guidelines.pdf.

Bailey, Z. D., Krieger, N., Agénor, M., Graves, J., Linos, N., & Bassett, M. T. (2017). Structural racism and health inequities in the USA: Evidence and interventions. *The Lancet, 389*(10077), 1453–1463. ISSN 0140-6736, https://doi.org/10.1016/S0140-6736(17)30569-X.

Begay, J. (2020, March 13). Decolonizing community care in response to COVID-19. Retrieved from: https://ndncollective.org/indigenizing-and-decolonizing-community-care-in-response-to-covid-19/.

Ben, J., Cormack, D., Harris, R., & Paradies, Y. (2017). Racism and health service utilisation: A systematic review and meta-analysis. *PLoS ONE, 12*(12), e0189900. https://doi.org/10.1371/journal.pone.0189900.

Copes, C. (2021). Can y'all please learn how to use "POC"? Medium.com. Accessed from: https://medium.com/an-injustice/can-y-all-please-learn-how-to-use-poc-f9931a31bcbc.

Goldberg, D. T. (Ed.). (1990). *Anatomy of Racism (Introduction)*. University of Minnesota Press.

Greenwood, B. N., Hardeman, R. R., Huang, L., & Sojourner, A. (2020). Physician–patient racial concordance and disparities in birthing mortality for newborns. *Proceedings of the National Academy of Sciences, 117*(35), 21194–21200. https://doi.org/10.1073/pnas.1913405117.

Marks, R., & Jones, N. (2020). Collecting and tabulating ethnicity and race responses in the 2020 Census. U.S. Census Bureau. Accessed from: https://www2.census.gov/about/training-workshops/2020/2020-02-19-pop-presentation.pdf.

McLaughlin, H. (2009). What's in a name: 'Client', 'patient', 'customer', 'consumer', 'expert by experience', 'service user'—What's next? *The British Journal of Social Work, 39*(6), 1101–1117. https://doi.org/10.1093/bjsw/bcm155

McWhorter, J. (2019, August 27). The idea that whites can't refer to the N-word. *The Atlantic.* Accessed March 25, 2020 from: https://www.theatlantic.com/ideas/archive/2019/08/whites-refer-to-the-n-word/596872/.

Nursing Council of New Zealand. (2011). *Cultural Safety, the Treaty of Waitangi and Maori Health: Guidelines for Cultural Safety.* Nursing Council of New Zealand, Wellington.

Office of Management and Budget (OMB). (1997). Revisions to the Standards for the classification of Federal data on race and ethnicity. Accessed from: https://www.govinfo.gov/content/pkg/FR-1997-10-30/pdf/97-28653.pdf.

Tello, M. (2017, January 16). Racism and discrimination in health care: Providers and patients. Accessed from: https://www.health.harvard.edu/blog/racism-discrimination-health-care-providers-patients-2017011611015. Harvard Health Blog, Harvard Health Publishing.

U. S. Census Bureau, (n.d.). Why we ask questions about place of birth, citizenship, year of entry. Accessed from: https://www.census.gov/acs/www/about/why-we-ask-each-question/citizenship/.

2

Culture-Focused Frameworks for Service Delivery

This chapter examines a variety of frameworks used to understand and address cultural issues in healthcare and human services. Frameworks in which to consider culture in the delivery of healthcare and human services have grown as culture is increasingly recognized as a determinant of health.

Cultural safety, as the focus, is discussed in more detail throughout the rest of this book. Other frameworks to gain prominence include cultural awareness, cultural sensitivity, cultural competence, cultural responsiveness and cultural humility. We provide a brief description of each framework as well as readings, activities, and case studies to apply from a professional practice standpoint.

Chapter Objectives

After completing this chapter, you should be able to:

- describe various frameworks for intercultural health and human service
- define and apply various frameworks to scenarios
- compare and contrast cultural safety with other approaches
- examine the relevance of cultural frameworks to your own practice.

Culture and Health

Far from being prescriptive and fixed, culture can include variables such as gender, age, religion, socio-economic status, ability, sexuality, and the ones mostly associated with cultural difference—those of ethnicity or race. So, what is the link between culture and health? Well, the link is significant.

Literature suggests that:

> Racial and ethnic minorities have higher morbidity and mortality from chronic diseases ... Among older adults, a higher proportion of African Americans and Latinos, compared to Whites, report that they have at least one of seven chronic conditions — asthma, cancer, heart disease, diabetes, high blood pressure, obesity, or anxiety/ depression. ... African Americans and American Indians/Alaska Natives are more likely to be limited in an activity (e.g., work, walking, bathing, or dressing) due to chronic conditions. (Ihara, n.d.)

But race or ethnicity alone does not explain disparities. Increasingly, psychologists and other health and human service professionals have recognized the importance of culture as an influence on health and social outcomes and by implication, on professional practice and service delivery.

Cultural awareness, cultural sensitivity, cultural competence, and cultural safety are some of the more established frameworks to influence services and health professional education. However, there is ongoing development and new modes of thinking as these concepts are applied and scrutinized. More recent frameworks arising from the U.S. include cultural responsiveness and cultural humility. A review of cultural safety in the U.S. found that while the term 'cultural safety' is not often used in the U.S., the tenets of cultural safety are practiced (Darroch et al., 2017). What is important always, is to find out about any local frameworks used within services and critique how well these can help meet the needs of local populations.

As cultures are diverse, so too are views about health and what it means to be healthy. The recent COVID-19 pandemic has illustrated this across a range of cultural groups. Health systems and human services that privilege a certain way of thinking unfortunately do this at the expense of others' ways of thinking and therefore at the expense of some people's health. With increasing emphasis on the rights of individuals to maintain their individual culture(s), providers and systems need to recognize that there is more than one way to do things and more than one belief system—there are many 'cultures', models, concepts, or frameworks.

In this chapter, we explore a number of these concepts and set the tone for how the rest of the book will unfold—firmly based within the framework of *cultural safety*. Of course, readers may have their own preferred or mandated frameworks for their work environment and that is fine. Before looking at the development of cultural safety and other rationales for its adoption, it may be useful to examine the historic developments that have led to what we have today.

Trans-cultural or Multicultural Practice

Although psychology has long acknowledged the importance of culture, it was the nursing profession in the U.S. that first firmly set its gaze on culture in practice. With the influx of European immigrants post World War II, differences between professionals and clients became more obvious.

The influence of anthropology was prominent in the 1960s with the ground-breaking work of nurse-anthropologist Madeleine Leininger, who pioneered the first real model of healthcare practice to incorporate cultural considerations. Trans-cultural nursing at that time focused on the importance of the healthcare professional to learn *about* cultural differences. Culture in this context, was a limited concept that related to ethnicity or race. Trans-cultural nursing practice involved developing the knowledge base of the nurse to incorporate certain cultural protocols toward clients of different ethnic or religious backgrounds.

Multicultural or cross-cultural psychology have had a similar history. Multicultural psychology has been defined as 'the systematic study of behavior, cognition, and affect in settings where people of different backgrounds interact' (Mio et al., 2020). Many textbooks for multicultural or cross-cultural psychology include chapters comparing racial or ethnic groups in terms of behavior, cognition, or affect (i.e., emotions) and even providing checklists of cultural differences for various groups such as Native Americans, Hispanics, Asian-Americans, Black Americans, Jewish-Americans, etc. Generally, those embracing the field of multicultural psychology or multiculturalism advocate for the maintenance and honoring of cultural differences between groups of people rather than assimilation, which we will learn about more in later chapters. Cross-cultural psychology often compares differences in psychological areas of interest between 'cultural' groups using statistical methods. Unfortunately, this approach tends to oversimplify both cultural variations, as well as psychological topics resulting in stereotyped oversimplifications that can potentially be more harmful than helpful.

One problem with trans-cultural nursing theory or multicultural or cross-cultural psychology, however, is the potential reliance on stereotyped notions of how an individual might behave based on ethnicity. Little attention is paid to life experiences and diversity within cultures, let al.one across cultures or, importantly, cultures that have been affected through colonization, dispossession, or forced migration. Imagine the usefulness of having care based on stereotypes of so-called 'American culture'. What exactly is American culture? If an American were in a hospital overseas, could they expect perhaps to be greeted with 'Hi y'all', or served a hot dog for lunch or would that be a very narrow stereotype with little relevance to yourself?

Trans-cultural, cross-cultural, or multicultural theories have been valuable in shifting from a homogenized mentality to one that is *regardful* of the individual needs of clients and communities. Trans-cultural nursing today, however, has grown and expanded, as evidenced by journals and professional societies related to this field. Other health disciplines and the broader field of human services are similarly responding to the recognition of the role of culture and cultural difference in professional practice.

> **Reading**
> Guilherme, M., & Dietz, G. (2015). Difference in diversity: Multiple perspectives on multicultural, intercultural, and transcultural conceptual complexities. *Journal of Multicultural Discourses, 10*(1), 1–21. https://doi.org/10.1080/17447143.2015.1015539.

Cultural Safety

Cultural safety will be discussed in more detail in the following and subsequent chapters. However, we need to establish an early understanding of this concept in order to compare and contrast other frameworks for intercultural practice. First, let's revisit the Nursing Council of New Zealand (2011, p. 7) definition of cultural safety, or *kawa whakaruruhau*:

> The effective (nursing) practice of a person or family from another culture, and is determined by that person or family. Culture includes, but is not restricted to, age or generation; gender; sexual orientation; occupation and socioeconomic status; ethnic origin or migrant experience; religious or spiritual belief; and disability.
> The (nurse) delivering the (nursing) service will have undertaken a process of reflection on his or her own cultural identity and will recognise the impact that his or her personal culture has on his or her professional practice. Unsafe cultural practice comprises any action, which diminishes, demeans or disempowers the cultural identity and well-being of an individual.

In short, the recipient of care determines whether the health professional or their service is culturally safe. Importantly, culture is defined broadly. It requires professionals to reflect on their own cultural identity and on their relative power as professionals.

Various approaches to health have viewed culture as a key determinant that can be 'managed' with increased cultural awareness or cultural competence on the part of providers. *Cultural safety* is one concept that the authors believe holds the greatest opportunity for transforming health practice in the U.S. and globally as it is one of the few frameworks that recognizes colonization, racism and discrimination as significant influences on health and social outcomes today.

We are not suggesting that an approach from New Zealand can simply be transferred to the U.S. context. The reason for considering its value in the U.S., is that it puts the onus for change on the service provider and system rather than on the client. It is an undertaking to think about the things that make us unique and to provide care that takes account of these differences. It is based on principles of professional practice rather than acquiring blocks of knowledge about cultures, which in a multicultural country such as the U.S., is expansive.

However, not everyone is ready to embrace the necessary elements of such a philosophy. We will discuss this further in later chapters that explore resistances to cultural safety.

Other Cultural Frameworks

We will now explore other frameworks that have focused on the issue of culture in healthcare and human services. Some of these overlap with cultural safety, and some have distinctly different goals. Various frameworks are not always well defined or have been defined differently by various writers. Overall, however, it is important to recognize that there are different terms and frameworks, and it is important to examine the aims and foci of the various approaches and their implementation in practice.

Cultural Awareness

Cultural awareness may be a framework that many have heard of or even participated in training. Cultural awareness training has been around for decades. It stems from anthropological studies of culture, which largely focused on racial or ethnic cultures, but more recently has included other forms of cultural difference. Cultural awareness is simply that—awareness of elements of culture—dress, foods, music, religious practices, rituals, social protocols, and so on. It's an important step for anyone working in an intercultural setting, but one which usually asks participants to look at 'the other'. It can lead to essentializing culture as something fixed and prescribed.

Cultural Sensitivity

Cultural sensitivity is perhaps less well-known as a framework, but more as a developmental consequence of cultural awareness training. Cultural sensitivity asks us to recognize our differences and accept others' right to those differences. In a sense, it requires us to accept that there are multiple worldviews, beliefs, and practices that everyone is entitled to hold and no one cultural group should be privileged above another. This is of course, easier said than done, as there are times when cultural practices and beliefs may clash with the current laws under which health professionals operate and this is the challenge of culturally safe practice to navigate these tensions.

Cultural Competence

Cultural competence originally developed in the U.S. and although in use across the country, it has been defined in many ways and used in many disciplines. Some definitions make it difficult to tease out the differences between cultural competence and cultural safety.

One definition of cultural competence is the ability of providers and organizations to effectively deliver health care services that meet the social, cultural, and linguistic needs of patients (Betancourt et al., 2002). A culturally competent healthcare system can help improve health outcomes and quality of care and can contribute to the elimination of *racial and ethnic* (emphasis added) health disparities (Ihara, n.d.). Strategies that may help achieve these goals include providing relevant training on cultural competence and cross-cultural issues to health professionals and creating policies that reduce administrative and linguistic barriers to patient care, including access to interpreters and increasing diversity in the workforce.

Another definition of cultural competence is 'the ability of systems to provide care to patients with diverse values, beliefs and behaviors, including tailoring delivery to meet patients' social, cultural and linguistic needs' (Betancourt et al., 2002, p. v). Campinha-Bacote (2002) defined cultural competence as a 'process, not an endpoint, in which the (nurse) continuously strives to achieve the ability to work within the cultural context of an individual, family, or community from a diverse cultural/ethnic background' (pp. 1–2). Cultural competence in some instances has been broken down to include clinical, organizational, and systemic cultural competence (DeSouza, 2008).

While there seems to be widespread adoption of cultural competence as a framework it has also come under much scrutiny and critique. It is often defined as the ability to work effectively with clients who are culturally different. The service provider is the focus in this definition. There is an emphasis on behavior or interactions that can be assessed as competent. But who decides whether a service provider's care or service has been 'competent'? What would this look like in practice?

Many of the social sciences have adopted the concept and terminology of cultural competence and expanded it to include elements which are, as you will see, similar to those employed in cultural safety. For example, cultural competence training in some psychology programs includes the importance of understanding the implications of a colonial history, notions of power (and disempowerment or empowerment), the consideration of how one's own culture impacts on their provision of care and how the care is received by clients. Side by side, it would be difficult to see any major difference between some ideas of cultural competence and cultural safety.

> **Readings**
> The following readings provide more details about cultural competence.
> Ihara, E. (n.d.). Cultural Competence in Health Care: Is it important for people with chronic conditions? Georgetown University, Health Policy Institute, Issue Briefs on Challenges for the twenty-first century: Chronic and Disabling Conditions, https://hpi.georgetown.edu/cultural/.
> Kohli, H. K., Huber, R., & Faul, A. C. (2010). Historical and theoretical development of culturally competent social work practice. *Journal of Teaching in Social Work, 30*(3), 252–271. https://doi.org/10.1080/08841233.2010.499091

Brach and Fraser (2000) provide some key strategies for improving the patient–provider interaction and institutionalizing changes in the healthcare system. These include:

1. Provide interpreter services
2. Recruit and retain minority staff
3. Provide training to increase cultural awareness, knowledge, and skills
4. Coordinate with traditional healers
5. Use community health workers
6. Incorporate culture-specific attitudes and values into health promotion tools
7. Include family and community members in health care decision-making
8. Locate clinics in geographic areas that are easily accessible for certain populations
9. Expand hours of operation
10. Provide linguistic competency that extends beyond the clinical encounter to the appointment desk, advice lines, medical billing, and other written materials.

Approaches that focus on increasing knowledge about various groups, typically through a list of common health beliefs, behaviors, and key 'dos' and 'don'ts', provide a starting point for health professionals to learn more about the health practices of a particular group. This approach may lead to stereotyping and may ignore variation within a group, however. For example, the assumption that all Latino patients share similar health beliefs and behaviors ignores important differences between and within groups. Latinos could include first-generation immigrants from Guatemala and sixth-generation Mexican Americans in Texas. Even among Mexican Americans, differences such as generation, level of acculturation, citizenship or refugee status, circumstances of immigration, and the proportion of his or her life spent in the U.S. are important to recognize.

It is almost impossible to know everything about every culture. Therefore, training approaches that focus only on facts are limited, and are best combined with approaches that provide skills that are more universal. For example, skills such as communication and medical history-taking techniques can be applied to a wide diversity of clientele. Curiosity, empathy, respect, and humility are some basic attitudes that have the potential to help the clinical relationship and to yield useful information about the patient's individual beliefs and preferences. An approach that focuses on inquiry, reflection, and analysis throughout the care process is most useful for acknowledging that culture is just one of many factors that influence an individual's health beliefs and practices. (Ihara, n.d.)

Activity

Ihara (n.d.) provides a number of strategies for improving the cultural competence of practitioners and organizations. Which strategies can you identify that are either already in place or would be beneficial in your local services? Choose one of the priority strategies for your location. If you had to write a proposal to your supervisor, how would you justify your request to implement your chosen strategy?

Cultural Humility

Cultural humility has arisen from the medical professions in the U.S. in response to what was seen as a limitation of cultural competence. *Culturally Connected* is a Canadian website that provides information and resources about cultural humility for health professionals. They define cultural humility using Tervalon and Murray-Garcia's (1998) definition:

- Cultural humility is a stance toward understanding culture. It requires a commitment to lifelong learning, continuous self-reflection on one's own assumptions and practices, comfort with 'not knowing', and recognition of the power/privilege imbalance that exists between clients and health professionals.
- A cultural humility approach is interactive: we approach another person with openness to learn; we ask questions rather than make assumptions; and we strive to understand rather than to inform.
- Embracing and learning about the similarities and differences between health professionals and clients, such as language, religious beliefs or values, age, gender, understandings of health and illness, or sexual orientation, can help providers to understand a client's health concerns, experiences, and preferences for care.

Reading

Gallardo, M. E. (Ed.). (2014). *Developing cultural humility: Embracing race, privilege and power*. Sage.

This book is a series of personal life experiences of psychologists from underrepresented communities and the challenges and rewards they experience in their own lives. The book is an excellent demonstration of how to examine and reflect on one's own cultural identity in very intentional ways.

Cultural Responsiveness

Cultural responsiveness is a concept that has been used in education and therapy. The concept has been applied to the work of school psychologists, teachers, therapists, social workers, occupational therapists, and even architects. The concept is not clearly defined and is lacking a strong literature base. The term seems to have been used interchangeably in the literature with other terms. Even so, we have included cultural responsiveness here should readers come across it in their own exploration of the literature or in their workplaces.

> **Reading**
> Below are a few readings relating to cultural responsiveness for those interested in exploring this area.
> Hays, P. A., & Iwamasa, G. Y. (Eds.). (2006). *Culturally responsive cognitive-behavioral therapy: Assessment, practice, and supervision*. American Psychological Association. https://doi.org/10.1037/11433-000.
> Misurell, J. R., & Springer, C. (2013). Developing culturally responsive evidence-based practice: A game-based group therapy program for child sexual abuse (CSA). *Journal of Child and Family Studies, 22*, 137–149. https://doi.org/10.1007/s10826-011-9560-2.
> Sisko, S. (2021). Cultural responsiveness in counselling and psychology: An introduction. In V. Hutton, S. Sisko (Eds.), *Multicultural responsiveness in counselling and psychology*. Palgrave Macmillan, Cham. https://doi.org/10.1007/978-3-030-55427-9_1.

Summary of Concepts

Overall, these various concepts or frameworks have provided us with evolving ways of thinking about and exploring culture, identities and diversity. The limitation of these frameworks or models is that we don't know very much about how they actually play out in practice. We don't have much research to show what works best or what actually makes a difference. The terms get thrown about as if they mean something in particular, but there are assumptions underlying what these concepts mean and major differences in how the concepts are defined, both within and between different groups.

If staff or students undergo some 'cultural' or 'diversity' training or workshops, what does that mean? What are they taught? How do we know it will make a positive difference? How do we know that what is taught is not harmful—perhaps creating more stereotypes or discrimination against certain groups?

While certain concepts, in an academic understanding, might be seen as more or less effective, when delivered in a workshop or similar it might depend on who was delivering the workshop, or how the issues are managed or presented. This makes it difficult to assess and understand exactly what is being taught and the impacts. We have therefore looked at each of the different concepts or frameworks and some of the weaknesses and strengths. Through this discussion and analysis, you should have a better understanding of how knowledge, values, and understanding influence practice.

Table 2.1 is a synthesis of some of the strengths and limitations of cultural safety and other frameworks. You might identify other strengths and limitations in your own analysis to add to this table:

Critical Thinking
- Reflect on the wide range of terminology and concepts relating to working in cultural contexts. Getting caught up in the current terminology can present a barrier for health professionals to working well in cultural contexts.
- How do professionals ensure that policies and frameworks for practice do not just linger in folders and on web pages of health services? What can you do as an individual to see policies put into practice?
- With many cultural frameworks, there is a strong desire to have a tool to measure outcomes. What is the risk of applying a tool that is developed by the service providers? How will you know if you have achieved competence, humility, or safety?

Table 2.1 Cultural frameworks, some strengths, and limitations

Framework	Key idea or elements	Strengths	Limitations
Cultural safety	– Be *regardful* of difference—treating people the same does not recognize or honor diversity – Decolonize practice: recognize the impact of colonizing history on current health, services, and systems – Recognize power relationships in practice – Reflective practice is a key tool to safety – Understanding own culture is key to recognizing its impact on others – Safety is determined by recipient of care	– Conceptually addresses elements that theoretically should improve health outcomes – Shifts power from providers to recipients – Shifts focus from the 'exotic other' to self – Is potentially applicable to any situation of cultural difference	– Requires more research – Has generally focused on application in interpersonal contexts and not as much in organizational or structural contexts – Resistance from some to concept of decolonization
Cultural awareness	– Focus on awareness of overt differences between groups – Stems from anthropology	– Provides a starting point to understand difference – Helps to establish basis for development of cultural safety	– Unachievable to be aware of or knowledgeable about all cultures – Based on anthropological overt differences – Views cultures as static – Can lead to stereotyping

(continued)

2 Culture-Focused Frameworks for Service Delivery

Table 2.1 (continued)

Framework	Key idea or elements	Strengths	Limitations
Cultural sensitivity	– Sensitive to elements of difference between self and clients – Recognizes rights to difference	– Extends awareness to an acceptance of the right to difference	– Improvement of practice requires more than sensitivity to issues – Stays at the individual level rather than organizational
Cultural competence	– Awareness, knowledge, and skills relating to culture Understand self as culture bearer – Recognition of historical, social, and political influences	– Relatively extensive literature base	– Potentially perpetuates colonizing practices and power imbalances – Can be deemed competent by other than recipients of care – not always consistently defined
Cultural humility	A commitment to lifelong learning, continuous self-reflection on one's own assumptions and practices, comfort with 'not knowing', and recognition of the power/privilege imbalance that exists between clients and professionals	Addresses the individual practitioner's potential power and privilege	Lack of literature

Making It Local

Find your current service's cultural framework. If you are a student, visit a health service in your local area. Critique the framework for how useful it would be in practice. Are there any particular frameworks that seem

> to be gaining prominence? If so, how are staff enabled or supported to implement these in practice?

Scenario
A local health service wanted to assess how well it was doing providing care to clients of a specific minority group: young, gay males 18–25. The practice manager developed a written client satisfaction survey that was left in the reception for clients to take and return to the receptionist.
- What do you think of this approach to assessing care for this population group?

As you answer, reflect on what assumptions you might have made about the practice manager, the receptionist, and the clients. It is natural to have some preconceived notions about who these people are, but it's also important to ask yourself, why? There is no right or wrong here—just encouragement to challenge our own, often unconscious biases. For example, who assumed the receptionist to be female? What might their religious background be if working in a clinic for gay men—can we really make any assumptions?

For all the information provided, it is really not possible to tell if this strategy would work or not. Cultural safety is about *how* you do something, not *what* you do. If the practice has established rapport with their clients, has identified that written surveys would be acceptable, possibly through asking their clients, and there is trust, then this could be a safe approach.

- How might you go about seeking feedback from clients? Would you use the same approach for all?
- How appropriate would this be in your specific location? Explain your response—why or why not?
- How would you personally know if you were providing culturally safe care to such a group?
- What potential biases might you have that could impact on your care of this demographic?

> **Further Reading**
> Walters, K. L., Johnson-Jennings, M., Stroud, S. et al. (2020). Growing from our roots: Strategies for developing culturally grounded health promotion interventions in American Indian, Alaska Native, and Native Hawaiian Communities. *Prevention Science 21*, 54–64. https://doi.org/10.1007/s11121-018-0952-z.
>
> Viruell-Fuentes, E. A., Miranda, P. Y., & Abdulrahim, S. (2012). More than culture: Structure racism, intersectionality theory and immigrant health. *Social Science & Medicine*.
>
> Wong, Y, J., McCullough, K., & Deng, K. (2019). Asian American Men's Health Applications of the Racial-Cultural Framework. In D. M. Griffith, M. A. Bruce, R. J. Thorpe, *Men's health equity. A handbook*. Routledge: New York.
>
> Peterson, L. S., Villarreal, V., & Castro, M. J. (2017). Models and frameworks for culturally responsive adaptations of interventions. *Contemporary School Psychology, 21*, 181–119. https://doi.org/10.1007/s40688-016-0115-9.

Conclusion

We have covered a variety of approaches to learning about and understanding cultures, identities and diversity in professional practice. We have not covered all the models and approaches to learning about these concepts. For example, diversity, equity, and inclusion training (DEI) is another approach that we have not covered but which you may want to investigate. Keep in mind that no single approach is likely to have all the answers. If there were such an approach, the health and social challenges facing us all in the U.S. would have been met and dealt with long ago. Cultural safety has arrived at a set of principles for ensuring that dominance, assumptions, and stereotyping do not result in a lack of safety and accessibility for those who have a different cultural background to the providers. In this way, it is not a discrete set of skills that we can perform to demonstrate safety, but rather a set of principles for practice that are relevant to any setting—including the need to ask or talk to those you provide care or service to, reflect on what you bring to the encounter, examine your own potential biases and assumptions, and decolonize practice.

This chapter has briefly explored frameworks that have been developed and used in health and other disciplines. While it may be an individual choice as to which framework resonates with readers, cultural safety is offered as the preferred approach because of its transferability across disciplines, contexts, and cultures and the essential element of recognizing the role of colonization in health outcomes today. This will be discussed in more detail in later chapters.

References

Betancourt, J. R., Green, A. R., & Carrillo, J. E. (2002). *Cultural competence in health care: Emerging frameworks and practical approaches* (Vol. 576). Commonwealth Fund, Quality of Care for Underserved Populations.

Brach, C., & Fraser, I. (2000). Can cultural competency reduce racial and ethnic health disparities? A review and conceptual model. *Medical Care Research and Review, 57*(Supplement 1), 181–217.

Campinha-Bacote, J. (2002). The process of cultural competence in the delivery of healthcare services: A model of care. *Journal of Transcultural Nursing, 13*(3), 181–184.

Culturally Connected. (n.d.). *Cultural humility.* https://culturallyconnected.ca/cultural-humility/.

Darroch, F., Giles, A., Sanderson, P., Brooks-Cleator, L., Schwartz, A., Joseph, D., & Nosker, R. (2017). The United States does CAIR about cultural safety: Examining cultural safety within Indigenous health contexts in Canada and the United States. *Journal of Transcultural Nursing: Official Journal of the Transcultural Nursing Society, 28*(3), 269–277. https://doi.org/10.1177/1043659616634170.

DeSouza, R. (2008). Wellness for all: The possibilities of cultural safety and cultural competence in New Zealand. *Journal of Research in Nursing, 13*(2), 125–135.

Gallardo, M. E. (Ed.). (2014). *Developing cultural humility: Embracing race, privilege and power*. Sage.

Guilherme, M., & Dietz, G. (2015). Difference in diversity: Multiple perspectives on multicultural, intercultural, and transcultural conceptual complexities. *Journal of Multicultural Discourses, 10*(1), 1–21. https://doi.org/10.1080/17447143.2015.1015539.

Ihara, E. (n.d.). *Cultural competence in health care: Is it important for people with chronic conditions?* Georgetown University, Health Policy Institute, Issue Briefs on Challenges for the 21st Century: Chronic and Disabling Conditions. Accessed from: https://hpi.georgetown.edu/cultural/.

Mio, J. S., Barker, L. A., Domenech-Rodriguez, M. M., & Gonzalez, J. (2020). *Multicultural psychology: Understanding our diverse communities* (5th ed.). Oxford.

Nursing Council of New Zealand (2011). *Cultural safety, the treaty of Waitangi and Maori health: Guidelines for cultural safety*. Nursing Council of New Zealand.

Tervalon, M., & Murray-Garcia, J. (1998). Cultural humility versus cultural competency: A critical distinction in defining physician training outcomes in multicultural education. [Editorial Research Support, Non-U.S. Government P.H.S. Review]. *Journal of Health Care for the Poor and Underserved, 9*(2), 117–125.

3

Cultural Safety

In this chapter, Cultural Safety, we describe the concept and the rationale for its preferred use as an underpinning philosophy and guiding principles for practice. The practice principles of cultural safety are discussed, including reflection on practice; the importance of communication and asking questions; consideration of power differentials; being mindful of how colonization impacts practice; racism and discrimination awareness and ensuring that professionals do not diminish, demean, or disempower others through their interactions.

This chapter will discuss cultural safety in more detail and explore the elements that make it a relevant approach for the U.S. health care and human services environments.

Chapter Objectives

After completing this chapter, you should be able to:

- define cultural safety
- describe the pathways to cultural safety

- identify the principles of culturally safe practice
- apply cultural safety to scenarios.

What Is Cultural Safety and What It Is Not

Cultural safety is both a philosophy and a way of working in professional health and human service settings. It is about ensuring that the cultural background of the professional does not dominate or put at risk the safety and well-being of any individual or group of a different cultural background to the professional. It is about *how* we do things, not just what we do.

Cultural safety is not about feeling guilty or believing any culture or cultural group is better than another. It is not a checklist for how to approach different groups. It is about becoming aware of one's own culture and understanding how it may interface with other cultures, with culture being more than race or ethnicity.

Why Cultural Safety as a Preferred Approach?

Cultural safety has been identified as a way of addressing social and health inequities, with its broader definition of culture than most other approaches that focus mainly on ethnicity or racial differences. It has arisen from an Indigenous perspective, from a country with a similar colonizing past to the U.S., which has demonstrated better outcomes are possible when there is the will (e.g., see Kurtz et al., 2018). Cultural safety is also relevant and beneficial to all participants in the healthcare experience, both clients and professionals delivering services.

Pathways to Cultural Safety

Some writers have conceptualized cultural safety as the third level in a set of three levels of cultural understanding (see Fig. 3.1). We, on the other hand, view cultural safety less as a hierarchy, but more like a continual

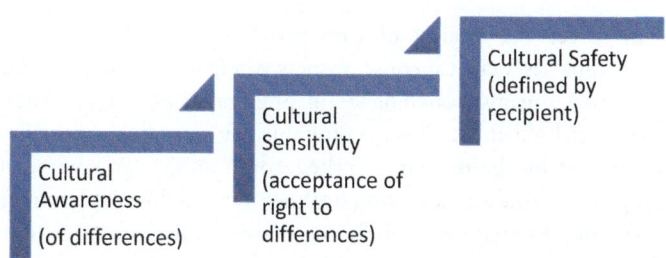

Fig. 3.1 Original stages of cultural safety as defined by Ramsden (Taylor & Thompson-Guerin, 2019)

process of reflection on and action applied to professional practice. First, let's review the levels of cultural safety as articulated in the New Zealand concept, before addressing more fully the application of cultural safety in practice.

The original stages of cultural safety, articulated by the late Irihapeti Ramsden, were transformative and had an impact that helped reshape nursing and midwifery education in New Zealand, Canada and Australia (Darroch et al., 2017). Sadly, this inspirational academic, whom one of the authors was fortunate to meet in the early days of cultural safety development, passed away before it could be seen where her work traveled. Ramsden (2002) was quick to acknowledge that the idea for cultural safety stemmed from a young Māori (the Indigenous people of New Zealand) midwifery student, who challenged the academy to think not only safety in terms of health and medical procedures, but in terms of culture. Others, such as Diane Wepa (2015), have taken on the further development and articulation of cultural safety. Curtis et al. (2019, p. 14) reviewed the literature around the concept of cultural safety and developed a new definition that makes the link to health equity more overt:

> Cultural safety requires healthcare professionals and their associated healthcare organisations to examine themselves and the potential impact of their own culture on clinical interactions and healthcare service delivery. This requires individual healthcare professionals and healthcare organisations to acknowledge and address their own biases, attitudes, assumptions, stereotypes, prejudices, structures and characteristics

that may affect the quality of care provided. In doing so, cultural safety encompasses a critical consciousness where healthcare professionals and healthcare organisations engage in ongoing self-reflection and self-awareness and hold themselves accountable for providing culturally safe care, as defined by the patient and their communities, and as measured through progress towards achieving health equity. Cultural safety requires healthcare professionals and their associated healthcare organisations to influence healthcare to reduce bias and achieve equity within the workforce and working environment.

A critical moment for the authors of this book came when Ramsden challenged non-Indigenous health professionals and academics to accept their own role in developing and implementing cultural safety. She suggested that cultural safety is everyone's responsibility and that it should not always fall to the members of the minority groups to explain their needs or adapt to the dominant cultures. Ramsden's message to the non-Indigenous audience was that the onus was on those in positions of power to examine their own cultures and seek to decolonize their engagements with those who differ in whatever aspect of culture.

In seeking to apply cultural safety in practice, we found that the cultural awareness stage really required an examination and understanding of our own cultures prior, and in addition, to developing awareness about others. We have chosen to make what was implicit in the original diagram more explicit in our model of cultural safety, shown in Fig. 3.2.

1. *Self-awareness*

Cultural awareness, usually considered the first step in the cultural safety literature, is about being conscious that there are differences between people. However, self-awareness may in fact be necessary in order to recognize our own individual culture(s). It is often not until we encounter someone from a different cultural background to ourselves that the influence of our own culture becomes apparent. For example, if you have been raised to view punctuality as a virtue, an important part of your core values, and you encounter someone for whom time is flexible, tension may arise. Imagine you have an appointment to meet

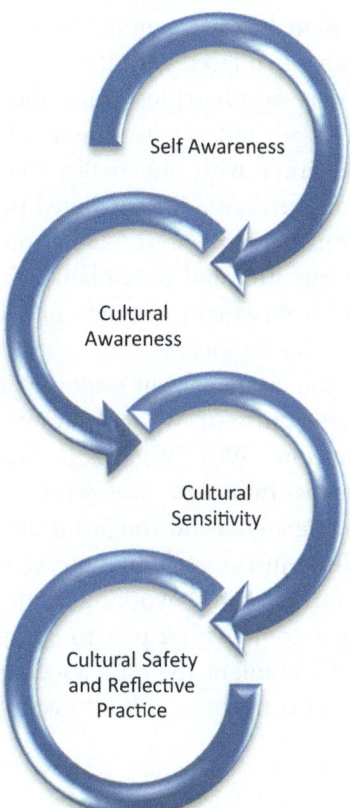

Fig. 3.2 An aspirational model of cultural safety—always incorporating new understandings and reflections to enhance culturally safe care, as defined by recipients (Taylor & Thompson-Guerin, 2019)

at 3:00 pm and your client arrives around 3.30, completely relaxed and unable to understand why you can't see them. How you respond will reveal much about the cultural interface. This doesn't mean there is no room to find common ground or that your needs have to be placed below those of the client's culture. It's how we arrive at that space that will determine the cultural safety of an engagement. Do you send them away because they 'missed' the appointment? Do you assume their lateness is a 'cultural thing'? How do you react when you are face-to-face with your late client—are you irritated or welcoming? Are you aware of your own reaction to the situation when faced with it?

There is no definitive answer here. Just think about the possible implications. If your client is late and you assume it is because their cultural background is less concerned with punctuality than you are—what are you engaging in? If you are even a little irritated by their lateness, what could be the impact on the encounter? Might you hurry things along, mindful of those coming after and potentially miss something important? What if they had been caught in traffic or even in a car accident? Would you have a different response?

The question is are you aware of your responses and where they come from? What presses your buttons? What makes you more or less likely to be patient with someone? Why? What is it about your own culture, identity or experiences that influence your own reactions? Cultural safety is not about saying anything goes and you just deal with it, but it is about making sure your culture just doesn't take precedence, because you are the one in the position of power. Working in the health and human services sectors does not come with a pass to engage in 'my way or the highway' philosophy. How might these interactions influence health or well-being outcomes and contribute to health equity, or inequities?

Activity

Take some time to reflect on your own culture:
- How do you feel about health? What is your own definition or understanding of health? Is health a personal responsibility or a communal one? Or is your health in the hands of a higher being? Who should be involved in your healthcare decisions—you and you only, or your extended family? Who do you want to be involved when discussing your own health?
- How do you show respect for authority? Do you look a person in authority in the eye or do you look down to show respect? How might you feel about someone who doesn't look you in the eye when speaking? What assumptions do you make about eye contact in communication?

- How do you feel about government involvement in your health? What role should the government have, if any? Explain your reasoning.
- How important is punctuality to you? From your perspective, what does it say about someone to be punctual?
- What is more important in your life—having a job and being financially secure or having good relationships with family and friends? Among your friends and family, how are these values expressed or experienced? What, if any, reactions do you have when coming in contact with others who may have differing values?

In answering these questions, it is likely that the answer to most of these may be 'that depends'. Context is important and you may find yourself moving along a continuum depending upon the situation. From a cultural safety perspective, it's necessary to know what biases, expectations, beliefs, and behaviors you are bringing into the encounter with someone who may hold different cultural perspectives, so as not to impose these on your client.

2. *Cultural awareness*

Cultural awareness, as already stated, is awareness of culture. The obvious or exotic differences are often easier to identify than the more subtle differences. These might include the mode of dress, foods people eat, or music preferences. However, cultural awareness also seeks to uncover the less obvious, including interpersonal behaviors, such as showing respect for authority by looking down, which may contrast with another culture that shows respect by looking directly at the person in authority as mentioned above. This could be a practice of some cultural groups, but of course, that doesn't mean every member of that group will display the same behavior, so cultural awareness learning is always to be taken with caution about applying such knowledge.

Cultural awareness is a stage that many people find very interesting and enjoyable and may include learning new words and protocols for interacting or communicating. These differences can be observed and enjoyed or visited for a period without requiring any fundamental change in practice or attitude. For some, it can be a little like going to a museum, but then you go home and continue to do things as you would before the visit. Indeed, many people experience cultural awareness when they go on a trip, maybe to another country. Unfortunately, many professional development workshops and educational settings tend to limit their cultural training to this stage of awareness. Cultural awareness also requires an understanding of one's own culture and the commonalities across all cultures that allow people to relate to and interpret any perceived differences.

Cultural awareness, simply put, is being aware that people are different. We discuss it again here because it is a widely used terminology, both within the domain of cultural safety as well as more generally. Cultural awareness is not entirely natural, it is not something that you are born with; awareness of differences between people is social and develops over time. If you watch small children, for example, two- to four-year-olds, they would generally not 'see' differences between people—kids are kids, grown-ups are grown-ups, and that's basically all they understand. Being aware that people are different is not problematic, but what is important is what you think of those differences and how you act on them.

For a long time, health professionals adopted the practice of treating everyone the same, intended to demonstrate a lack of prejudice on the part of health services and professionals. However, evidence has suggested that disparities in health and social outcomes of some populations can be attributed in part to cultural differences between clients and care providers. Increasingly, people began talking about the need to be 'culturally aware' and not assume everyone belongs to a homogenous base, that everyone is coming from the same position.

Cultural awareness approaches often focus on learning about the things that make cultural groups different from one another, while overlooking many of the features in common. While a useful first step, learning these sorts of details can also lead to stereotyping and inappropriate behavior or interactions. It is not possible to learn everything there is to know about all the cultures that you encounter in your professional practice or your life and experience. This is also why the cycling between cultural awareness and self-awareness is so critical. There is an old saying that if you are pointing the finger at someone, there are three pointing back at you. When we only focus on 'the other' and their cultural 'ways', we tend to see them as exotic and different, but fail to see how they are also human variations. When we look at ourselves (three fingers pointing back at you) and engage in self-awareness and see how we ourselves are culture-bearers, we can understand the complexity, nuance, and fluidity of cultural identities. Cultural safety principles provide a useful addition to your knowledge base as they can be applied to any point of 'perceived' difference between you and those in your care, including age, socioeconomic status, genders, abilities, religions, or sexualities.

3. *Cultural sensitivity*

Cultural sensitivity is intended as the next step up from cultural awareness. It means being sensitive to the differences learned about through cultural awareness. Sensitivity assumes that professionals can apply their awareness of cultural differences to their own practice. Cultural sensitivity validates the right to difference. Article 22 of the Universal Declaration of Human Rights states that:

> Everyone, as a member of society, has the right to social security and is entitled to realization, through national effort and international cooperation and in accordance with the organization and resources of each State, of the economic, social and cultural rights indispensable for his dignity and the free development of his personality. (United Nations, 1948)

Cultural sensitivity is also thinking about your own attitudes and beliefs and how they might affect the person you are working with, as well as taking into account the cultural issues that might influence your clients.

In this step you might say, 'OK, there are cultural differences, and now I can be sensitive to those differences. As a professional, I can consider different modes of operating for my clients'. Difference is legitimated—difference is OK—and it is about being sensitive to the possibility that my difference might impact on others. In this stage, the professional reaches an understanding that individuals are entitled to hold differing worldviews, values, knowledge, and beliefs. It should not be a matter of leaving these cultural foundations at the door in order to access care. The professional needs to be sensitive to differing needs and expectations, and work to accommodate these where possible. It is not and should not be the goal to 'convert' or 'colonize' someone to your preferred culture. This is challenging when certain experiences conflict with your personal beliefs and values.

Cultural safety does not ask you as the professional to change any of these aspects—you have just as much right to your culture as those you seek to provide service to—but what is important is that in choosing a service career, you are not trying to diminish, demean, disempower, or impose your views on another. You may have strongly held views about abortion, for example, but in providing professional care to another, these should not come into the engagement with a client. Indeed, for culturally safe practice, you need to be well aware of how your views may harm the outcomes for your client if you do not manage it. If this is untenable to you as an individual, you may have to think about your career choices, as the professional role is about providing judgment-free, culturally safe care. This is absolutely essential for health and outcomes to improve.

There is recurring debate in this country about the 'right to discriminate' on the basis of 'religious protection'. On a personal level, that is something for an individual's conscience. In health and human service provision, however, think about what this actually means. Look at the following scenario:

> **Scenario**
> Two women bring a baby to the local clinic. The staff member asks the mother to complete the paperwork. Both women put their name on the form, only to be told that the clinic would need to know who the 'actual mother' was.
> - What message has the couple received from this interaction?
> - Whose construct of family is being privileged?

- What are the potential risks to the baby and parents of this experience?
- How might a professional manage their personal belief system when encountering someone with different beliefs?

Sensitivity is also about being sensitive to elements of racism, discrimination or othering. Intent is not enough to guard against a client experiencing racism, discrimination or feeling 'othered'. If the women took offense at the question about who is the 'actual' mother and the professional stated, 'Oh, I don't have a problem with same-sex couples. I have friends who are gay', does this make a difference? The women may have experienced the comment as insensitive and discriminatory regardless of the intent of the staff member.

Mistakes are often unavoidable, but how they are managed reveals much about character and safety. Reflection in and on practice is a necessary tool to achieve cultural safety. So rather than being anxious about making a mistake, think about how this might have been done differently. Let's accept there was a 'clinical' reason for asking such a question—perhaps a hereditary concern, for example. A more culturally sensitive approach would be to preface any such question with an explanation: 'I just need some background information that could be relevant, would you mind specifying who is the birth mother?' Unless there is a rationale for the question, it has the potential to demean the family, whether intended or not. And, if a mistake or a potentially insensitive comment or question is made, then, acknowledge it, apologize, and demonstrate actions for reparations or changing behavior.

4. *Cultural safety*

Irihapeti Ramsden (2002), who spearheaded the original cultural safety movement in New Zealand, believed that it was not enough to focus on the 'exotic' aspects of an individual's or group's culture as was often done in cultural awareness, cultural sensitivity or trans-cultural nursing approaches. In contrast to trans-cultural nursing, which originally sought to describe and respond to the cultural differences, cultural safety involves recognition of power imbalances and historical, political, social, and economic structures. Cultural safety requires the health professional (or others) to understand their own culture and to acknowledge the power imbalance brought about by dominant systems. It requires professionals to actively seek to ensure no 'cultural harm' is done through actions that may impact on clients.

Cultural safety has gained momentum in places like Canada and Australia, with a growing body of literature challenging existing approaches to health and social care for Indigenous and other peoples. It is important to acknowledge that the cultural safety framework itself came from Indigenous Peoples. However, rather than suggest simply applying a foreign concept to an American context, it is obvious that without some adaptation and regard of local contexts, histories, and worldviews, this act itself would be an unsafe one. While cultural safety is an Indigenous construct, it requires the dominant or colonizing culture to engage in processes of self-reflection and decolonizing practice that ultimately has relevance for any client.

Examining the New Zealand experience suggests that clinical competencies, technical expertise, and theoretical knowledge form only part of the care equation when the recipients of care differ in some way from the professional. For example, a health professional may have the technical skills to administer a vaccine, may know vaccination guidelines and timeframes, and may be very knowledgeable about the diseases that are prevented through vaccination programs. But what skills are required when trying to administer a vaccine to a four-year-old who is very distressed or when working with a family who may have good reasons to distrust or be skeptical about vaccinations?

Although cultural safety has arisen from the disciplines of midwifery and nursing, other health disciplines as well as social and human services have found or are finding relevance for their practice. Even where other philosophical frameworks have emerged, there can be no denying that the New Zealand experience has had a profound influence in focusing on culture and colonization in health. There are numerous readings and resources that might be examined for a deeper understanding of the development and conceptualization of cultural safety.

> **Readings**
> To learn more deeply about these topics, the following readings are a good place to start:
>
> Irihapeti Merenia Ramsden's PhD thesis: '*Cultural Safety and Nursing Education in Āotearoa and Te Waipounamu*' (2002) is available online through Massey University, New Zealand.
>
> Browne, A., Varcoe, C., et al. (2009). Cultural safety and the challenges of translating critically oriented knowledge in practice. *Nursing Philosophy, 10*(3), 167–179.
>
> Curtis, E., Jones, R., Tipene-Leach, D., et al. (2019). Why cultural safety rather than cultural competency is required to achieve health equity: A literature review and recommended definition. *International Journal of Equity in Health, 18,* 174. https://doi.org/10.1186/s12939-019-1082-3
>
> Smith, S. (2012). *Cultural safety in nursing education: Increasing care for LGBT individuals.* http://hdl.handle.net/2376/3442. Washington State University, Master of Nursing. https://research.libraries.wsu.edu/xmlui/handle/2376/3442

Cultural Safety Principles

The following is a brief summary of the principles of cultural safety, adapted from the Nursing Council of New Zealand (2011):

1. The need for health and human services professionals to *reflect on their practice* is a critical aspect of culturally safe practice. As most health and human service professionals are members of dominant cultural groups, think about how this might impact on clients who are members of minority groups. Remember too, that dominant and minority are relative terms. For example, women are not necessarily a minority but have specialized healthcare needs that can render them a 'vulnerable' group in certain contexts.
2. *Talk, ask, engage in dialogue with the client.* This might seem obvious. Yet there are countless examples of encounters where clients are

spoken about, around, and on behalf of, but often not talked to or with. (See the chapter *Intercultural communications*). A culturally safe approach will require true engagement with the client to understand their unique needs, beliefs, understandings, and preferred ways of doing things. Where there is a perceived or actual barrier to discourse (or conversation), clients can remain un-engaged and un-empowered in response to their own health care or other needs. Talking, asking, and engaging with the client is not always easy to achieve so this topic will be discussed further in later chapters.

3. *Seek to minimize the power differentials between yourself and your client.* Western healthcare and human services have traditionally been hierarchical in nature, although this is slowly changing. Professionals may be wittingly or unwittingly in positions of power over their clients. What might shift the power balance in your professional practice setting? Language is a very important indicator of power in healthcare. Think about the way in which clients are sometimes referred to as 'non-compliant', 'absconder', or 'frequent flyers'. These kinds of labels position the professional as the one in power, whereas the clients are reduced to simple labels.

4. *Undertake a process of decolonization.* This was a somewhat controversial aspect of the cultural safety model that was criticized in the press in New Zealand and Australia, countries with more recent colonizing histories than the U.S. It is this element, however, that separates cultural safety from all other approaches. The original concept of cultural safety involved acknowledging the key role of a colonizing history in contemporary health and social outcomes for Indigenous Peoples specifically. While the colonizing experience of New Zealand differs somewhat from that of the U.S. (see the chapter on global issues for details), we examine what a decolonizing process may mean in a U.S. setting.

5. *Ensure that you do not diminish, demean, or disempower others through your actions.* Sometimes it is easier to identify culturally unsafe practice than it is to identify culturally safe approaches. Both, however, require a level of self-awareness and a willingness to critique practice and systems. Actions can include subtleties of body language, how

you say things and what you say, as well as more overt behaviors. We provide numerous examples throughout this book.
6. *Undertake to examine your own and others' potential for racism, discrimination, stereotyping, or othering.* Understanding racism and discrimination involves realizing how these are experienced by those on the receiving end—not about an individual's intent. It is not enough to declare that we are not 'racist' or 'sexist' or 'homophobic' or any other discriminating label if the person we engage with is experiencing our interactions as such. Interrogating our assumptions and being mindful of the tendency to view people as 'the other' are all principles that can be applied to professional practice.

Critical Thinking

What are some fundamental differences between New Zealand and the U.S. that might make the transferability of cultural safety more challenging?

The New Zealand state nursing exam has included questions focusing on cultural safety. What do you think of this idea for the U.S.? How would it be received locally for psychology and other health or human service professionals? What are the arguments for and against?

In 2015, the MCAT, the exam for entrance to medical school, added a new section, the Psychological, Social and Biological Foundations of Behavior, which requires an understanding of cultural and social differences, social stratification, and access to resources, and factors that influence communication and behavior. Indeed, concept 9 of this section relates specifically to cultural and social differences and how they relate to well-being (see the Association of American Medical Colleges, n.d., for more information).

There remains no single, standardized, or universally accepted model of cultural education for settings outside of New Zealand. In the absence of a fully articulated, locally relevant and universally accepted philosophy, cultural safety has been examined for its relevance to the U.S. and other healthcare and human services settings. It is a concept that is yet to be fully considered for its appropriateness in the U.S. context. Review the following scenarios:

> **Scenario**
> An elderly veteran was called to a clinic to collect their new hearing aid. They have lost or broken several in the past. On arrival the receptionist said in front of a waiting room of other people: 'Now (name), how many is this? You can't keep getting them replaced you know. You better look after this one!'.
> The veteran was furious at the treatment. They turned and walked out without the hearing aid.
> - What elements of culturally unsafe practice can you identify?
> - What cultural differences might have influenced their response?
> - What role, if any, should the receptionist have in commenting on a client's reason for attending?
> - What may have caused them to leave the clinic without being seen?
> - How would you try to make this a culturally safe encounter for the elderly veteran?
> - As you read the scenario, did you imagine a particular gender for the receptionist and the veteran? What might this say about unconscious bias?

> **Scenario**
> A young couple, still in their teens, has been asked to sign consent for a major operation for their child. Both seem unwilling to sign anything. Some staff are suggesting involving Child and Youth Services if they won't sign. They are, after all, putting their child at risk by delaying surgery. The doctors have already spoken to the parents and have now requested nursing staff to do what they can to obtain consent. The mother signs the form but then both parents leave their child in the hospital and return home.
> Using the principles, answer the following:
> 1. Reflection on practice. How would you feel about your practice if you were involved in the above scenario?
> 2. Who has the power in this scenario? What pressures are brought to bear to obtain consent? Even though consent has been obtained, has it been done in a culturally safe manner? If not, why not?

3. What dialogue could have been engaged in with the parents? Would you have involved anyone else—if so, who and why?
4. What aspects of this encounter might be considered as colonizing in nature? How might you decolonize this scenario?
5. What may have been behind the responses? Are there possible cultural issues resulting in the parents' reluctance? You might need to investigate local cultural norms for child rearing, roles, and responsibilities.
6. How might this have been managed differently? What evidence is there that this family may have been demeaned, disempowered, or diminished?
7. Does the context make a difference in this scenario? If so, in what ways does it make a difference? What needs to be taken into account?

Looking at the above, it is important not to apply the same expectations to everyone in order to be equal and reasonable. For the young parents (any parents), depending on individual circumstances, they may have been reluctant to sign a consent form because of cultural considerations, or simply because of past experiences or any number of other possible explanations. European or White Americans for example, may expect biological parents to be the ones responsible for providing consent for their children. Biological parents are therefore naturally the first ones spoken to about their children and the first ones from whom information is sought. However, not all cultures, and therefore, not all White or European people, construct parental responsibility in the same way.

Some cultures hold biological parents responsible for nurturing and care, but also share the responsibility with others in their kinship systems for major decision-making. Therefore, without consideration of the potential for a different set of needs, treating this young family the same as everyone else might not in fact be equal. It could have put them in an untenable situation from which they felt compelled to leave. They may simply have wanted other family there to help make the decision. Perhaps both had jobs they needed to go to and could not afford to lose. That is not to say that these are the case in every situation. However, these are things to be examined in context. Rather than compel someone to consent, asking questions such as, 'Is there anyone else we can contact to help you right now?' or instead of judging the actions, or make assumptions, greater effort could have gone into talking about the parents' reluctance.

> Health and human services professionals may not know, and not need to know, what is behind the preferences and decisions of clients and communities in order to be culturally safe. They simply need to be aware of the right to be different, and to respect the right to one's own worldview and cultural values.

Making It Local

Think about also the transferability of cultural safety principles to clients who differ from health and human service professionals in other ways—either by religion, gender, socioeconomic status, abilities, sexuality, or age.

Do you have any particular groups within your local area that may also require care that is regardful of certain differences? Who are these groups? How might their 'cultural differences' need to be incorporated into their care? For example, is there a large aging population or LGBTQ community in your region? Do some staff have unexamined, negative attitudes toward older or LGBTQ people that might affect the care provided? What about rural populations? There is research to suggest that some rural-backgrounded people may delay seeking health care because of a cultural mindset that prioritizes their work over their own health, for example. Of course, this could equally apply to others on the basis of economics, gender, or other influences, but what is important is to recognize any reaction you might have to specific cultural groups and ensure that any negative biases or assumptions do not impact on care provided.

What is the demographic makeup of your community and what might this mean for shaping practice or preparing for practice?

Conclusion

In this chapter, we have identified cultural safety as a useful framework for examining and critically reflecting upon practice. This text does not seek to provide a prescriptive approach to the care of clients of a differing background to the health professional. Instead, it is hoped that students and health professionals will develop a set of culturally safe principles for practice; examine previously held knowledge, beliefs, attitudes, and understandings; and develop readily transferable skills for practice in any setting.

References

Association of American Medical Colleges. (n.d.). *Psychology, social, and biological foundation of behavior section: Overview.* https://students-residents.aamc.org/applying-medical-school/article/mcat-2015-psbb-overview/.

Curtis, E., Jones, R., Tipene-Leach, D., et al. (2019). Why cultural safety rather than cultural competency is required to achieve health equity: A literature review and recommended definition. *International Journal of Equity and Health, 18*, 174. https://doi.org/10.1186/s12939-019-1082-3.

Darroch, F., Giles, A., Sanderson, P., Brooks-Cleator, L., Schwartz, A., Joseph, D., & Nosker, R. (2017). The United States does CAIR about cultural safety: Examining cultural safety within indigenous health contexts in Canada and the united states. *Journal of Transcultural Nursing: Official Journal of the Transcultural Nursing Society, 28*(3), 269–277. https://doi.org/10.1177/1043659616634170.

Kurtz, D. L. M., Janke, R., Vinek, J., Wells, T., Hutchinson, P., & Froste, A. (2018). Health sciences cultural safety education in Australia, Canada, New Zealand, and the United States: A literature review. *International Journal of Medical Education, 9*, 271–285. http://dx.doi.org.ezaccess.libraries.psu.edu/10.5116/ijme.5bc7.21e2.

Nursing Council of New Zealand. (2011). *Cultural safety, the Treaty of Waitangi and Maori health: Guidelines for cultural safety.* Nursing Council of New Zealand.

Ramsden, I. (2002). *Cultural safety and nursing education in Aotearoa and Te Waipounamu.* University of Wellington.

Taylor, K., & Thompson-Guerin, P. (2019). *Health Care and Indigenous Australians: Cultural safety in practice* (3rd ed.). Red Globe Press. ISBN-13: 9781352005424.

United Nations. (1948). *Universal Declaration of Human Rights* (United Nations General Assembly in Paris, General Assembly Resolution 217 A). https://www.un.org/en/universal-declaration-human-rights/.

Wepa, D. (Ed.). (2015). *Cultural safety in Aotearoa New Zealand* (2nd ed.). Cambridge University Press. https://doi.org/10.1017/CBO9781316151136.

4

Models of Health and Well-Being

The majority of health and human service professionals in the U.S. subscribe to a biomedical model supported by their training and an historical dominance of this approach. Yet, it has become apparent that outcomes in health and human services are not fully explained or addressed by biomedicine alone. This chapter describes various models and definitions of health and how they fit within the context of diverse and complex client care.

Chapter Objectives

After completing this chapter, you should be able to:

- discuss the various definitions of health and articulate a personal definition of health
- compare and contrast various models of health
- critically analyze the implications of competing or complementary models of health for healthcare or human services practice

© The Author(s), under exclusive license to Springer Nature Switzerland AG 2021
P. B. Thompson and K. Taylor, *A Cultural Safety Approach to Health Psychology*, Sustainable Development Goals Series, https://doi.org/10.1007/978-3-030-76849-2_4

- examine the role of health and human services professionals in relation to various models of health.

Definitions of Health

If you were asked to explain what it is that makes a person healthy, you might suggest things like eating healthy food, maintaining good hygiene, getting plenty of exercise and rest, not smoking, and so on. Or would you? If you were a person who believed strongly in a biomedical definition of health, you might. However, another person might say that what makes them healthy is having family around, breathing fresh air, feeling as if they 'belong'—knowing who they are and where they come from. This would be a different way of thinking about being healthy, and there might be as many ways of thinking about health as there are people reading this book.

> **Activity: Personal Definition of Health**
> What do you do to stay healthy? There would obviously be many different ways to answer this question. Take some time before you continue reading to write down your own definition of health. You will need to revisit this as we discuss various models of health to see where you are most closely aligned.

Regardless of your views of health, as professionals, much weight will undoubtedly be placed on Western biomedical models of health care—and that's OK. That is your training and the service in which you might practice. You are not asked to take on your clients' health beliefs or their preferred way of living, but you are asked to provide care that doesn't diminish or demean another because of them. No one needs to negate their own culture and cultural values in order to practice cultural safety principles and appreciate another's culture. The precepts of cultural safety simply ask all health and human service professionals to *reflect* on their own culture and *acknowledge* the potential impact that differing ways of knowing and power relationships might manifest. Cultural safety asks you to act with care, compassion, and courage as you attempt to meet the health and social care needs of people in your care.

Not everyone shares the same ideas about what health means or what illness means. These different understandings lead to, for example, differences in what people will do to be healthier or what they do when they are ill, and what sorts of things might be prioritized. Perhaps the most cited definition of health is the World Health Organization (WHO, 1978) definition:

> Health is a state of complete physical, mental, and social well-being and not merely the absence of disease or infirmity.

This is the definition in the Preamble to the Constitution of the World Health Organization adopted by the International Health Conference, New York, 19–22 June 1946 (Official Records of the World Health Organization, no. 2, p. 100) and entered into force on April 7, 1948. *It* came about partly in reaction to ideas of health as being *not ill*—ideas that lead to healthcare practice being focused on simply treating disease or illness.

The WHO definition might seem like a pretty good one at first glance, but what is 'complete' and who decides if someone is healthy or not? If someone has a disability, are they not healthy? What if someone has a disease or chronic condition such as asthma—are they not healthy or 'well'? What is well-being? Who defines well-being? Taken literally, the WHO definition would suggest that none of us is ever really fully 'healthy' or 'well'. Indeed, consider that nearly half of the U.S. population have at least one chronic disease (Raghupathi & Raghupathi, 2018) and about 1 in 4 adults live with a disability (CDC, n.d.).

Let us look at other ways to define health. Indigenous definitions often view health as being more than an absence of disease—health requires a physical, spiritual, mental, and emotional well-being of *whole communities* and usually contains a connection to the land or sea and the environment. For example, the United Nations (2016, p. v) provides this definition of health: 'the right to health materializes through the well-being of an individual as well as the social, emotional, spiritual and cultural well-being of the whole community'.

> **Website**
> Explore the U.S. National Library of Medicine website *Native Voices: Native Peoples' Concepts of Health and Illness* for a wide range of sources and information relating to health and wellbeing and Native Peoples.
> https://www.nlm.nih.gov/nativevoices/index.html

> **Reading**
> Koithan, M., & Farrell, C. (2010). Indigenous Native American healing traditions. *The Journal for Nurse Practitioners: JNP*, 6(6), 477–478. https://doi.org/10.1016/j.nurpra.2010.03.016
> https://www.ncbi.nlm.nih.gov/pmc/articles/PMC2913884/

One important difference in the Indigenous definition is the focus on the health of the 'whole community' as compared to the WHO definition, which focuses on 'individual' health. While this difference might seem minor, it has huge implications for healthcare funding, healthcare practice, and how 'health' is measured. If we were to look at how a whole community was faring, for example, if we saw high rates of crime and unemployment as well as high rates of various health conditions such as obesity and diabetes, we might have a very different approach to helping that *community* become healthier. These arguments warrant consideration of models of health, which influence such issues as funding allocation (structural dimensions) or health care and other human services practice.

Elements of an Indigenous definition of health can be challenging if you view health as only being located in the body. Spirituality is generally not something people can see or put a finger on—it is not something you can touch. Land, on the other hand, is something we can see and touch; but relationship with land and its importance to health and well-being generally don't feature in Western models of health—not overtly at least. Yet, spirituality can and does play a role for many non-Indigenous people as well, even though it may not be prominent in Western health. And with that, let us now look at the different models of health.

Models of Health

As students or employees in the health and human services professions, you signal your alignment to particular models and definitions of health and practice. The model to which the majority of health professionals will subscribe in the U.S. today is a Western biomedical model. There will be a diversity of approaches within this model, with some practitioners also incorporating social models and other definitions of health along a spectrum. For example, integrative medicine is a more holistic approach to health and illness that is growing in popularity. Often, the health model that we function under is not obvious or explicit, but it does influence our professional practice. This may not present any problems or issues for us professionally until we work with clients who have a different understanding or worldview about health; it is then that it becomes important to reflect on and be aware of health models and understandings.

Western medicine has much to offer. Few could argue with the benefits and progressions made in disease treatments, trauma management, and public health for example. However, Western medicine is based upon a particular worldview that is not universally accepted. Within the biomedical model, health is viewed through physical changes to an individual's body. Western medicine sees the body as an entity of interrelated systems that requires a state of homeostasis for optimal functioning. Health is mostly about anatomy and physiology, with disease transmission based on germ theory.

The biomedical model has been criticized for being reductionist—reducing health and illness down to the smallest biological elements; mechanistic—assuming that diseases have a primary biological cause;

dualistic—neglecting social and psychological influences; and empirical—assuming that causes of all illness can be objectively and biologically identified (Lyons & Chamberlain, 2006). Additionally, the biomedical model has been criticized for being overly disease focused (at the expense of health), and overly interventionist and intrusive (Lyons & Chamberlain, 2006). We can't be too critical, however. The biomedical model has an important role to play but can be enhanced by fusion of approaches that allow for diversity both at the individual and broader population level.

In contrast to the biomedical model, a social model of health explores the causes of inequality between groups, such as racial or ethnic groups or groups with differing economic status. In a social model of health changes are made through public policy to improve health-related living and working conditions. The social model of health underlies social and economic determinants of health. Social and economic status (SES) is a statistical measure that classifies individuals, households, or families according to income, occupation, and education. This area of research shows that the wealthier you are, the higher your job status, and the higher the level of education you have achieved; the longer you will live, the less illness you will suffer and, if you do become sick, the better the quality of treatment you will receive and, therefore, the better your health outcomes will be (for example, see Marmot, 2015). Table 4.1 shows some key differences between the biomedical model and the social model of health in terms of focus, assumptions, key indicators, causes, interventions, and goals.

The 'biopsychosocial' model of health falls between the biomedical model and the social model if we were to think of these models as falling on a continuum, rather than as discrete models. Engel proposed the biopsychosocial model in 1977. In this model, biological, psychological, and social elements are considered to be influencing factors in health. Some have suggested that the biopsychosocial model is really the biomedical model in disguise (Lyons & Chamberlain, 2006). Other concerns with the biopsychosocial model include that the different elements and how they differ from one another have not been clearly defined. That is, how is 'social' different from 'psychological', or how is 'psychological' different from 'biological'?

Table 4.1 Key differences between biomedical and social approaches to health

Element	Biomedical	Social
Focus	Individuals who are sick	Social groups' living and working conditions
Assumption	Individual responsibility for health	Social responsibility for health
Key Indicator	Individual pathology	Health inequalities between social groups
Causes of Illness	Gene defects; Micro-organisms (e.g., viruses) Lifestyle: risk-taking	Political & economic factors (e.g., poverty) Cultural factors (e.g., discrimination)
Intervention	Cure individuals who are sick; Modify behavior of individuals at risk	State intervention to reduce inequalities Community participation
Goals	Cure disease Preserve life Reduce risk factors to prevent disease in individuals	Prevent illness Ensure quality of life Reduce health inequities between social groups

Source Adapted from Germov and Poole (2007)

What is the impact of health care that is at odds with, or perceived as being at odds with, your own personal set of beliefs and values? Balance—whether it is physiological or otherwise—would seem to be a core value of most cultures' ideas of health and well-being.

Health professionals today often refer to 'evidence-based practice'. Evidence-based practice is an approach to health care and human services work that assumes that there is evidence available upon which care should be delivered and that, if we just follow the evidence, then our practice will be effective. The problem with the approach of evidence-based practice is that these assumptions limit what is accepted as evidence. For example, the 'evidence' is based on Western biomedical notions that are reflected through the use of randomized control trials (RCTs), held up as the gold-standard of medical research (Ezzy, 2002). However, RCTs often fail to take into account the social and other elements influencing health and illness or that those methods can be inadequate to identify such elements. Additionally, consider that many Indigenous Peoples and other long-standing health practices such as Traditional Chinese Medicine or Ayurvedic medicine have thousands of years of evidence-based practice on which they have developed their own particular health strategies and wisdom. This kind of knowledge, in a Western evidence-based notion, is often undermined and determined to be lacking in evidence because these practitioners have not followed the Western research paradigm and yet, increasingly, there is a re-orientation happening toward non-Western knowledges and cultural practices to deal with environmental and other health concerns.

Despite not being fully accepted in Western medical and health systems, complementary and alternative medicines have increased in popularity. These approaches reflect the reality of multiple bodies of knowledge and evidence throughout the world and over time. However, look at the language used to describe approaches that fall outside the dominant biomedical model. Healthcare practices used by millions of people for generations are deemed to be 'complementary or alternative'. This has implications for funding, health insurance, and uptake, with most clients 'funneled' into mainstream systems and services. Pharmaceutical industries are invested in research that reinforces health behaviors that demand a prescription rather than research that supports advice to engage in relaxation techniques, eat a balanced diet, and exercise more.

Film and Website of Interest

Escape Fire: The Fight to Rescue American Healthcare is a 2012 film by Matthew Heineman and Susan Froemke that explores the problems with the American healthcare system and provides some direction for an improved healthcare system that is focused on prevention and healing.

The interactive website http://www.escapefiremovie.com/ provides a wealth of activities, information, and tools for gaining a better understanding of the issues and solutions to improved health care in the U.S.

Making It Local

> - What health or related services can be found in your local area? Who are the main users of these services?
> - Are there any that would fall under the category of 'complementary or alternative'?
> - Who uses these services?

Social Determinants of Health

The Social Determinants of Health (SDoH) are gaining greater prominence as it has become clearer that biomedicine does not fully explain or deal with causation, behaviors, health seeking practices, or outcomes. We discuss this idea more fully in the Determinants of Health Chapter, but we introduce it here as it is an important concept in understanding different ways to think about health and illness. The Office of Disease Prevention and Health Promotion defines the social determinants of health as the:

> …conditions in the environments in which people are born, live, learn, work, play, worship, and age that affect a wide range of health, functioning, and quality-of-life outcomes and risks. Conditions (e.g., social, economic, and physical) in these various environments and settings (e.g., school, church, workplace, and neighborhood) have been referred to as "place." In addition to the more material attributes of "place," the patterns of social engagement and sense of security and well-being are also affected by where people live. Resources that enhance quality of life can have a significant influence on population health outcomes. Examples of these resources include safe and affordable housing, access to education, public safety, availability of healthy foods, local emergency/health services, and environments free of life-threatening toxins. (Office of Disease Prevention and Health Promotion, n.d.)

In the U.S. today, it seems that a lot of people have concerns with what is perceived to be *socialism*, when what is actually being put forward is a means of addressing inequities. Social models of health promote an equitable approach to health and social care, to make it affordable, accessible, and acceptable to all. The COVID-19 pandemic meant people became acutely aware of their own vulnerabilities and potential for getting sick despite all efforts to 'protect' themselves. In this context, most people understood the value of health care being accessible to everyone.

> **Activity**
> Look up definitions of socialism; universal health care; Affordable Care Act; privatized health insurance; single-payer versus multi-payer health care. Write down what you see as the pros and cons of each.

Primary Health Care

Primary health care (PHC) was first put forward as a somewhat radical approach aimed at addressing the inequities in health among the world's populations. PHC, like cultural safety, is both a philosophy and a model of service delivery. The U.S. is a nation with major disparities in health among its populations. The Bureau of Primary Healthcare committed to adopt a PHC approach to health care in the 1970s. Again, like with cultural safety, PHC is yet to be fully implemented. 'Health for all by the Year 2000' was a catch-cry of much of the 1980s and 1990s, and yet PHC still remains a distant aspiration or a service model only for underserved or marginalized populations. What has happened is that the catch-cry simply gets updated—it was to be by 2020, now it is to be 'by 2030' and undoubtedly the goalposts will continue to shift. So, what is PHC and why should we bother with it?

Primary health care outlined a set of principles for health service delivery that was believed to have particular relevance for the world's Indigenous Peoples and others in less developed countries. The U.S. is a highly developed country, where much of Western health care focuses on high-technology, high-cost, curative and treatment interventions. However, in developing countries, where health infrastructure and health needs are far more basic, this kind of health care generally has little relevance. In the U.S. however, some sectors of the community experience health outcomes that are similar to outcomes within poorer countries.

> **Websites**
>
> See the World Health Organization website for Primary Health Care including the 2019 Fact Sheet: https://www.who.int/news-room/fact-sheets/detail/primary-health-care.
>
> This webpage hosted by the Commonwealth Fund provides an excellent and engaging overview of primary health care for women: Transforming Primary Health Care for Women Part 1: A Framework for Addressing Gaps and Barriers (Zephyrin, Suennen, Viswanathan, Augenstein, & Bachrach, 2020: https://www.commonwealthfund.org/publications/fund-reports/2020/jul/transforming-primary-health-care-women-part-1-framework.

At the World Health Organization Conference held in the Russian city of Alma-Ata in 1978, the following definition was developed and presented within the Declaration of Alma-Ata to which the U.S. became a signatory:

> Primary health care is essential health care based on practical, scientifically sound and socially acceptable methods and technology made universally accessible to individuals and families in the community through their full participation and at a cost the community and country can afford to maintain at every stage of their development in the spirit of self-reliance and self-determination. It forms an integral part both of the country's health system, of which it is the central function and main focus, and of the overall social and economic development of the community. It is the first level of contact of individuals, the family and community with the national health system bringing health care as close as possible to where people live and work and constitutes the first element of a continuing healthcare process. (*Declaration of Alma-Ata*, WHO, 1978)

This is not the complete definition, but rather the core components that are often repeated when trying to succinctly describe PHC:

- essential (or first-level care)
- accessible—available to the people wherever they are, with no barriers to using the service
- acceptable to the people—there is no conflict with the manner in which services are delivered, that is, it is culturally safe to use the service as provided
- full participation—it is not top-down directed care
- affordable—it does not rely on high-cost, highly technologized treatments and interventions.

> **Critical Thinking**
> How does the PHC model fit in with the clinical or other professional practice you have experienced so far? Or how does the PHC model fit with your experience of healthcare services?
>
> Would you say the health service provided was universally accessible, acceptable, and affordable? Why or why not? What changes would need to be made to make it accessible, acceptable, and affordable? (You may want to revisit your definitions above about various health policies.)

> **Reflection**
> You are walking by a river when you see someone in the middle, drowning. You jump in and rescue them. You commence basic life support, and they are OK. Before you go any further, there is another person. The same thing—you save them, treat them, and then can't get any further down the river, because the tide of people falling into the river continues.
>
> It's a seemingly endless cycle—drowning, rescue, save, treat. While you are so busy saving everyone, you are fast becoming exhausted, unable to continue to meet the needs of the people in the river for much longer. With your attention so firmly focused on saving each person you come across, there is no time to move upriver to see what is causing all of these people to be in the river in the first place.

> This old analogy is used to illustrate the difference between the various levels of health services—tertiary, secondary, and primary. With the focus so firmly on treatments and intervention, the problems become self-perpetuating. Nothing is being done to stop the problems before they occur (i.e., prevention). All levels of health services are important, but when one is given more resources and support than other levels or when the various services work in isolation rather than collaboration, then 'health for all' is impossible.

The Principles of Primary Health Care

PHC requires healthcare services to re-orient away from high-cost, technology-driven curative models to a focus on prevention and promotion. What follows is a brief overview of some key tenets of primary health care.

1. *A social view of health*

The social view of health recognizes that health is more than just the absence of disease and infirmity or the prevention of individual and family health problems. It is the recognition that providing a safe environment—such as clean air, adequate water, and sanitation supply, sound occupational health and safety standards, acceptable standards of housing, the lowest possible levels of poverty—is also vital. It is a fact that in the U.S. today, not all sectors of the community enjoy such basic rights as these. We can look at the alarming rates of skin infections leading eventually to an epidemic in renal failure among Indigenous Peoples, but if we fail to take a social view of health that accepts the root causes as having more to do with injustice and inequality than medical and behavioral factors, the impact of our practice will be limited. For health and human services professionals specifically, it means incorporating a wide range of interventions that recognize the person as a whole in the context of their lives, families, communities, and culture.

Holistic care is not new—it just remains something that is often given more lip service than practical application. Increasingly, there is greater attention in research and literature to the social determinants of health. Biomedical approaches that do not include the social determinants are limited in their potential to effect better health outcomes.

2. *Focus on self-reliance*

The individual, family, and community need to participate in defining the health problem. That is, they must set what the health priorities are for them, their family, and community. They need to be supported by funding and resources to determine the strategies to counter these problems. Historically, too many approaches have tended to develop dependency rather than self-reliance.

How important is the principle, 'focus on self-reliance', in light of past policies that actively promoted dependence and took away individual control?

3. *Multidisciplinary team approach*

Traditionally doctors, nurses, and other health professionals have been the dominant holders of power once a person entered the healthcare system. PHC requires the power to be located with the consumer and that all people—professionals, service providers, support staff, family, and the individual—actively participate in decisions about health issues in the community. In a PHC approach, the multidisciplinary team is meant to include more than the immediate members of a health center or unit. They need to coordinate care with professionals who may be geographically distanced from the clients. Podiatrists, occupational therapists, dental therapists, social workers, psychologists, etc., all need to be recognized as part of the multidisciplinary team in a PHC approach rather than as discrete service providers. The silo mentality that has been fostered by mainstream health service structures often stifles efforts to provide a truly comprehensive PHC approach, and clients can easily 'fall through the cracks'.

4. Diversity of workforces and practitioners

In an Indigenous context, PHC cannot be adequately implemented without Indigenous health personnel across all areas and levels of the health service. This principle applies more broadly as well. Women's health, Veterans' health programs, LGBTQ health, rural initiatives, all benefit by having workforces that are representative and have knowledge of their communities. If members of your own cultural group are not visible in a specific setting, how effective can that service be in truly understanding the needs of the population being served?

> **Activity**
> Look at the diversity in your own workplace or in your experience of health services. How representative are the staff for the population they serve?

5. Focus on main needs as defined by the community

The issue here is of utilization of resources that will benefit the greatest number of people. This means that, rather than powerful lobby groups determining where the health dollar is spent, priorities include the most common issues and areas of concern.

In order for this to happen, however, people need access to information in a way that is meaningful to them, which is discussed in Intercultural Communications. Making informed decisions about health and well-being can be limited by poor communications, misunderstandings, and low levels of health literacy.

Additionally, for health services to meet the needs of the community requires a certain level of engagement with the local community. When communities are engaged in their healthcare services there are many benefits such as improved health outcomes, improved equity, improved access to services, services are more relevant and acceptable, the quality is enhanced as well as responsiveness (Bath & Wakerman, 2015).

6. Special attention to high-risk and vulnerable groups

PHC must not only address the major and most common health problems in our society but must also pay special attention to those groups in our society who are high risk, vulnerable, and very often voiceless against the continuous lobbying of the more powerful groups. The demands of social justice are that these groups—women, people in remote areas, and people with disabilities—are assisted with affirmative action strategies to improve their health status. PHC is about addressing disparities, particularly disparities within already high-risk groups. One of the challenges in focusing on specific groups, if it is not done following a comprehensive PHC approach, is the risk of further marginalizing or relocating the vulnerability.

7. Individual and community participation

This is, arguably, one of the more important principles of PHC. It means allowing people, no matter where they are—in the Intensive Care Unit in the most technologically sophisticated hospital in the country or living in the middle of the desert—to be in control of their health care, in fact, of their life. It means genuinely encouraging individuals and communities to define their own needs and ways of meeting those needs. This is probably the hardest issue for health professionals to face because of the misconception that 'we have the knowledge, the expertise. We know best. Trust us!'.

Scenario

A client has refused a blood transfusion. You have been asked to explain to the client the consequences and your supervisor has asked you to 'Make sure you get the consent signed'.
- How do you respond in this situation?
- What principles of cultural safety could you apply here?
- What would you do if a client or community made decisions that you did not believe were in their best interests?

> Does locating the control with the individual and community mean that health professionals merely have to go along with whatever is required, or do they have a role in ensuring that the choices made are truly informed by the provision of accessible information?
>
> - By talking with the client, in the scenario above, you find out that their objection is not on religious grounds but based on a fear of needles. How might this change what you do?
> - What would you see as a culturally safe outcome in both situations—fear of needles or religious objection?
>
> PHC is most often thought of as an approach that occurs outside of hospital settings, but the principles of participation in decision-making are just as relevant in any healthcare or human services.

8. *Broad range of strategies*

PHC includes services and strategies that meet acute needs. Rehabilitation and long-term care also come under the PHC banner, as does political action to create conditions that are conducive to, and that create and maintain, healthy environments. PHC, as with cultural safety, is not about *what* you do but *how* you do it. Once again, it is about attitudes.

9. *Prevention*

As integral to PHC as the strategies above are, one strategy that is often associated most clearly with PHC is prevention. Substance misuse, motor vehicle accidents (MVAs), poor living conditions and overcrowding resulting in respiratory disease, chronic infections, and communicable diseases account for a majority of preventable impairments. Any treatment or rehabilitation service that does not address the issue of prevention is of little value.

One of the major challenges with prevention is that of readiness to change. How many people do not actually engage in preventative health care until they have had their first health scare? Prevention is a difficult concept to embrace for anyone who feels relatively well and is unable to see the potential harm in their actions.

10. *Inter-sectoral collaboration*

This principle rests on the recognition that the conditions for health are determined beyond the healthcare system. Inter-sectoral collaboration means cooperation and coordination across government and non-government departments. When health is thought about in its social, cultural, economic, political, and environmental context, as well as in its medical context, factors such as housing, employment, town planning, education, and motor vehicle design have to be taken into consideration.

More than 40 years since the Declaration of Alma-Ata, it is not unreasonable to wonder where that commitment has gone. For a developed nation, the healthcare needs of the majority of our population are dramatically different from those in underdeveloped and developing countries. Health challenges facing those in Third World regions have largely been met here in the U.S. through stringent public health measures and infrastructures that are not yet realized in other parts of the world.

PHC was in recognition of the fact that major inequities have existed and continue to exist, even in developed countries. PHC was promoted as a means of addressing these inequities and of meeting future challenges. Since Alma-Ata, there have been several developments and redefinitions of PHC.

Activity

Find a current definition of PHC. How does this differ from 'primary care' and 'public health'? Critique services that describe themselves as PHC to see how they match the original principles. How do the principles of PHC and cultural safety relate? Are there any commonalities?

Activity
Look at these websites for their relevance to PHC:
- Bureau of Primary Health Care https://bphc.hrsa.gov/
  https://bphc.hrsa.gov/about/what-is-a-health-center/index.html
- The American Academy of Family Physicians, Health Care for All: A Framework for moving to a Primary Care-Based Health Care System in the United States: https://www.aafp.org/about/policies/all/health-care-for-all.html
- Centers for Medicare and Medicaid Services Patient's Bill of Rights: https://www.cms.gov/CCIIO/Programs-and-Initiatives/Health-Insurance-Market-Reforms/Patients-Bill-of-Rights

Readings
Birn, A. E. (2018). Back to Alma-Ata, from 1978 to 2018 and beyond. *American Journal of Public Health, 108*(9), 1153–1155. https://doi.org/10.2105/AJPH.2018.304625
  https://www.ncbi.nlm.nih.gov/pmc/articles/PMC6085028/
  Rifkin, S. B. (2018). Alma Ata after 40 years: Primary health care and health for all-from consensus to complexity. *BMJ Global Health, 3*(Suppl 3), e001188. https://doi.org/10.1136/bmjgh-2018-001188. Accessed from: https://www.ncbi.nlm.nih.gov/pmc/articles/PMC6307566/

Making It Local
- Explore the websites for health services within a defined geographic region, not just your local community. Does your county have a Board of Health? Look at the website for information on health services and the approach to health care and health services.
- What, if any, PHC services exist in your city or town or region or county or state?

> • What evidence is there of PHC principles being applied in non-PHC settings?

There is no doubt that excellent professional skills are essential for practice in all settings. However, no matter how good your skills, without a reorientation of health services and practices that incorporate a PHC approach, professionals will be destined to provide band-aid solutions at best. In an environment where the 'photo opportunity' can drive political activity, few politicians would be as happy to cut the ribbon on a basic water supply to a community as they would open yet another hospital. Health professionals and services need to shift their focus to genuine primary health care that reflects the commitment previously made by our politicians and that is reaffirmed by current health initiatives.

Health Beliefs and Models of Care

While mainstream health services in the U.S. are dominated by a biomedical approach to health, we have already noted that not everyone holds the same perspective. There are many other specific beliefs about health and illness causation. Germ theory, for example, may not be part of these beliefs.

Remembering that people are diverse in their cultural beliefs and practices, and are influenced by differing life experiences, we cannot provide a succinct discussion of health beliefs and how these might impact upon care. However, there are some excellent readings on the beliefs of different cultural groups that provide some insight into what could be influential for some clients. From a cultural safety perspective, it is not necessary to even know what these health beliefs could be, only that clients may not subscribe to the same explanations and practices as you might. The following scenario looks at the role of health professionals when faced with conflicting health beliefs and models of care.

> **Scenario**
> The community you are working with has high rates of smoking and chest infections. You want to conduct community education sessions, but no one attends, except for one elderly person who tells you that the community's health problems are all related to the buffalo being absent from their lands.
> - How do you respond to this information?
> - How might you have approached your practice differently?
> - What role might you have in supporting the community to address the elder's concern, if any?
> - What happens to your concerns about smoking rates and chest infections? Do you just forget about them? What would you do differently?
>
> As we can see, health is very much culturally determined. More often than not, professionals dismiss Indigenous and other explanations because of their supposed lack of 'scientific credibility'. This is understandable. Most people will value their own culture and beliefs above others. It is the extent to which this occurs that can be problematic. If we place our own culture as 'superior to' rather than as simply 'different from' another, then we engage in ethnocentrism—a destructive attitude that has the potential to cause harm.

> **Scenario**
> A child in the hospital has not been improving and is eventually moved to the Pediatric Intensive Care Unit (ICU). The family is increasingly concerned and calls for a traditional healer to attend their child. The healer examines the child and identifies that his spirit has 'jumped out' of his body and it has to be retrieved.
>
> > How would you respond to this explanation of the child's deteriorating health?
> >
> > What would you see as your role in this encounter?
>
> **Activity**

> Can you think of any incident in your own experience that radically altered your own long-held views and beliefs?

People throughout history have demonstrated considerable expertise and resilience in adapting to new situations. The introduction (or imposition) of Western health care has not been rejected. On the contrary, many non-Western people view Western medicine and treatments as useful adjuncts to their own healthcare practices. So, the challenge for professionals is to find a way to incorporate and accommodate multiple views and conceptualizations of health without positioning one at the expense of another.

> **Activity**
> Ideas about health and illness change over time. What do you believe about health and illness today?
> - Review how you personally define health. Has anything changed for you since the earlier exercise?
> - Is your definition related in any way to your culture?
> - Has your way of thinking about health changed over time?
> - Think about your own worldviews and cultural values. Whose cultural values and worldviews are often prioritized or reflected in healthcare services that you are familiar with?

> **Film**
> The film *Wilhemina's War: Fighting HIV and AIDS in the South*. PBS, Independent Lens: https://www.pbs.org/independentlens/films/wilheminas-war/. Depicts the variety of concerns to be considered when working in some communities. This film shows issues of stigma, barriers to accessing care, issues with health literacy and prevention, and extended family and community dynamics relevant to health and care. This film

> also looks at how policy decisions impact on delivery of health care and services.

Conclusion

This chapter explored a selection of models for health care, including PHC as a model with the potential for providing culturally safe and accessible care. It is extremely important not to assume a standard set of beliefs and preferred ways of operating for any particular group. Cultural safety requires health and human service professionals to ask the individual how they might want to be cared for. This is a challenge in itself, but a necessary undertaking in achieving positive health outcomes for recipients of care, especially where there is a cultural difference between provider and recipients.

References

Bath, J., & Wakerman, J. (2015). Impact of community participation in primary health care: What is the evidence? *Australian Journal of Primary Health, 21*(1), 2–8. https://doi.org/10.1071/PY12164.

CDC. (n.d.). *Disability impacts all of us.* https://www.cdc.gov/ncbddd/disabilityandhealth/infographic-disability-impacts-all.html.

Ezzy, D. (2002). *Qualitative analysis: Practice and innovation.* Allen & Unwin.

Germov, J., & Poole, M. (2007). *Public sociology: An introduction to Australian society.* Allen & Unwin.

Lyons, A. C., & Chamberlain, K. (2006). *Health psychology: A critical introduction.* Cambridge University Press.

Marmot, M. (2015). *The health gap: The challenge of an unequal world.* Bloomsbury.

Office of Disease Prevention and Health Promotion. (n.d.). *Social determinants of health: Overview.* https://www.healthypeople.gov/2020/topics-objectives/topic/social-determinants-of-health.

Raghupathi, W., & Raghupathi, V. (2018). An empirical study of chronic diseases in the United States: A visual analytics approach. *International Journal of Environmental Research and Public Health, 15*(3), 431. https://doi.org/10.3390/ijerph15030431.

United Nations. (2016). *The state of the world's indigenous peoples.* https://doi.org/10.18356/7914b045-en. https://www.un.org/development/desa/indigenouspeoples/wp-content/uploads/sites/19/2018/03/The-State-of-The-Worlds-Indigenous-Peoples-WEB.pdf.

World Health Organization. (1978, September 6–12). *Declaration of Alma-Ata.* Paper presented at the International Conference on Primary Health Care, Alma-Ata, USSR. http://www.who.int/publications/almaata_declaration_en.pdf.

5

History Taking

We discuss the importance of understanding history in healthcare and human services work in this chapter. We will address how historical relationships, policies, and events relate to health and well-being and to health and social disparities in the U.S. today. This chapter includes descriptions of past practices that are not only known to be unethical by any standard but proven to have had a detrimental effect on the health and well-being of subsequent generations.

Chapter Objectives

After completing this chapter, you should be able to:

- identify historical events and influences that manifest through the health of communities and individuals today
- describe some of the policies, laws, and other government actions that impacted health and well-being of various groups
- understand the intergenerational impact on contemporary health

- critically analyze the role of health and human service professionals in implementing policies and practices that had harmful impacts on health.

History and Health

No health professional would or should think about trying to care for a client without first obtaining an adequate history. If asked, most people may be able to rattle off what they believe are major health concerns facing our nation and specific communities. Most often, however, they are citing *symptoms* or *consequences* of *historical impacts* on successive generations. Before being able to deal with current health issues, it is necessary to look at what has contributed to the current health crises facing our country today.

Health and human services professionals understand that a crucial step in providing good care to a client is to obtain an adequate history. Obtaining a history is more than just documenting a client's health history or their experiences. The person who we see and experience in front of us carries with them their own experiences as well as those experiences of family and others in their communities. Historical events, whether they be political, social, environmental, economic, or personal, have irrevocably changed the health and well-being of people and communities. Health and human services professionals will be limited in the safety of care they can provide until we can critically examine our nation's history and the impact it has had on health and well-being.

W. E. B. DuBois wrote in *Black Reconstruction in America*, 'We have too often a deliberate attempt so to change the facts of history that the story will make pleasant reading for Americans' (1935). Learning about the history of colonization and the impacts can be confronting, especially for people who find themselves living in reasonable comfort and privilege. There can be reluctance for some to engage in what may be seen as 'dwelling on the past.' Yet in a professional setting, professionals must inform themselves of the issues that have led someone to need their services. In this sense, taking a 'history' is part of professional responsibility. Taking a history can also be rewarding, as it adds capacity to both the provider and recipient of care and contributes to relationship and rapport building.

But how far back should we go when we explore history? Certainly, the consequences of colonization are continuing to be revealed in the health and social status of today, and this is evident globally. So do we need to know all that history? Let's look briefly at why colonization has been so significant to health outcomes today.

Relevance of History

Few people would deny that European connections with this land that some had known as *Great Turtle Island* are brief in comparison to those of the first inhabitants. It is estimated that Indigenous Peoples have lived in this land that we now call the U.S. for *around 15–20,000 years*. The earliest evidence of human habitation, earthwork mounds, have been found around what is now the Mississippi River and have been estimated to have been built around 4500 BC. How long have non-Indigenous people—mostly Europeans—lived in the U.S? Most people cite 1492 as the defining year of when Europeans first arrived in North America with the arrival of Christopher Columbus. When represented visually as years on the timeline in Figure 5.1, the comparison is dramatic. Can you see the European section? It hardly shows up. What does this timeline mean to the inhabitants of the U.S. today?

As we think about our 'history taking' and its role for us as professionals, we need to go all the way back to the early colonization of the U.S. and understand how those early relationships started. With any relationship, the foundation is key to understanding how those relationships developed and came to be what they are today. The Doctrine of Discovery was the premise, or ideas, that formed the basis of a series of decrees or papal bulls in which Christian domination was justified during the fifteenth century. For example, in 1493, Pope Alexander VI issued a papal bull *Inter Caetera*, in which the Pope authorized Spain and Portugal to colonize, convert, and enslave the Native peoples of the Americas and to enslave Africans (National Library of Medicine, n.d.a). The English Translation of the Spanish 1513 *El Requierimento* for King

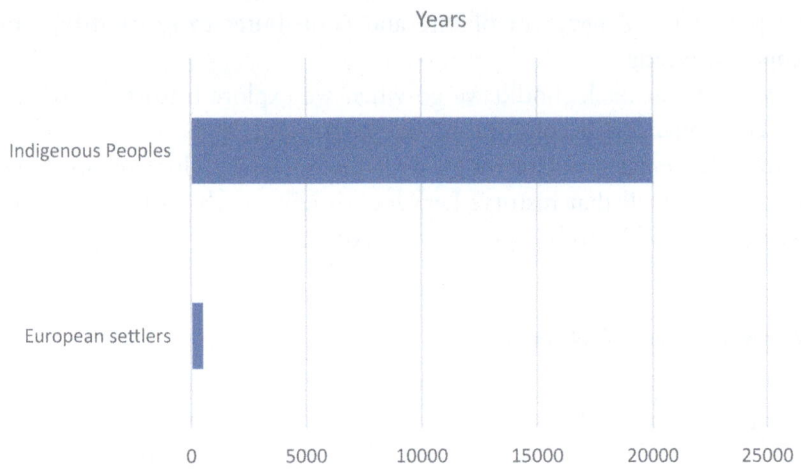

Fig. 5.1 Indigenous and European occupation of *Great Turtle Island*, now called the U.S.

Don Fernando and his daughter Doña Juana, Queen of Castille and León shows the blatant demand of Christian domination and the effects of not agreeing:

> Wherefore, as best we can, we ask and require you that you consider what we have said to you, and you take the time that shall be necessary to understand and deliberate upon it, and that you acknowledge the Church as the ruler and superior of the whole world, But if you do not do this, and maliciously make delay in it, I certify to you that, with the help of God, we shall powerfully enter into your country, and shall make war against you in all ways and manners that we can, and shall subject you to the yoke and obedience of the Church and of their highnesses; we shall take you, and your wives, and your children, and shall make slaves of them, and as such shall sell and dispose of them as their highnesses may command; and we shall take away your goods, and shall do you all the mischief and damage that we can, as to vassals who do not obey, and refuse to receive their lord, and resist and contradict him: and we protest that the deaths and losses which shall accrue from this are your fault, and not that of their highnesses, or ours, nor of these cavaliers who come with us. (National Library of Medicine, n.d.b)

> **Scenario**
> Someone comes into your house one day and tells you that you must agree that their beliefs are better than yours and that therefore they are the rulers and 'superior of the whole world'! And that if you do not agree, they can take whatever they want from you and do whatever they want to you, including enslaving you or even killing you and all your family and loved ones, and should any of that happen, it will all be your fault! In this scenario, we also need to understand that these people coming into your home do not speak the same language as you, so, you're not even sure what they are saying.
>
> Does any of that sound familiar?
>
> Can you see any parallels to some of our current cultural tensions?
>
> What about the victim-blaming at the end of this statement: that whatever happens will all be 'your fault'? Does that sound like anything we see today? Think about some common reactions under circumstances of rape or police brutality when victims are often blamed for what happened. Health conditions today, despite being known to be influenced by a range of social determinants, are also often blamed on those who are experiencing them.
>
> Imagine what it might be like to experience this, and what effect it might have on you. You might say, 'well, they wouldn't get into my house in the first place,' but they do get in and you don't have a chance or the resources to stop them, because they outnumber you and your family. Can you imagine going through all the grief processes as your way of life erodes before your eyes? How long might it take you to 'get over it'?
> Consider that this may be what many Indigenous peoples continue to experience—deep, unresolved grief and loss.

Let's revisit that timeline. Based on time alone, Native American ownership, or sovereignty over the land, should be indisputable. The Doctrine of Discovery, more aptly described as the Doctrine of Domination (Newcomb, 2008), and the concept of *terra nullius* were the doctrines that justified European claim to lands around the world. These ideas were grounded in notions that non-Christians were less than human and provided Europeans with the legal, religious, and political justification for colonization, enslavement, and seizing land. Not only was ownership disputed, but the very existence of an entire group of people was ignored. *Terra nullius* literally means 'land belonging to no-one.' Think about the consequences of this beginning to all relationships and interactions that have followed between those doing the dominating and those being dominated. From the perspective of *terra nullius* , the people who were here were basically made to be invisible; that they didn't even exist, indeed, that they didn't matter. Today, we see vast amounts of literature in areas such as 'social inclusion,' 'anti-racism,' and social movements such as Black Lives Matter, aimed to improve health, social, and well-being outcomes that can be connected to these early ways of thinking and interacting.

Part of the Doctrine of Discovery included the enslavement of people to make colonization possible. This included the enslavement of the people on their own lands, as well as the bringing of enslaved people from other lands. Understanding contemporary issues in health and well-being in the U.S. requires the knowledge of the history of enslavement and its part in the colonization of North America. Enslavement, domination, and displacement define much of the history from the fifteenth century. While many cite 1619 as the beginning of slavery in the U.S., others cite 1526 as a more accurate date when a Spanish ship of enslaved Africans arrived in what is now South Carolina (Guasco, 2017). That group of Africans rebelled, and the Spanish could not maintain their settlement. These early events of rebellion are a too often silenced part of history.

By today's understandings it may be hard to imagine the overt dismissal and dehumanization of entire populations, but these ideas continue to inform laws and policies that maintain domination over the land and people. Understanding the circumstances surrounding the colonization of the U.S. is essential to have some sense of the prevailing worldviews underpinning these events. This is not only necessary for the anticipated number of readers who have not grown up in the U.S., but also for those whose educational experience in the U.S. provided little other than a Eurocentric, or 'white-washed' view of colonization. It is a sad indictment of the U.S. school system that many students even today remain unaware of our own history beyond a one-sided view of European 'discovery,' 'exploration,' and 'settlement.' 'Recent surveys, however, show that young people in America have enormous gaps in what they understand about the history of slavery in this country. According to a 2018 report from the Southern Poverty Law Center, only eight percent of high-school seniors surveyed were able to identify slavery as the central cause of the Civil War. Two-thirds of students did not know that a constitutional amendment was necessary to formally end slavery' (Smith, 2020).

In this book, we cannot fully address the imbalance, other than to provide a cursory review of colonization as it related to the U.S. experience and the relevance of this today for healthcare and human services. To develop culturally safe professionals, we encourage extensive and regular study of history to inform understanding that will benefit your professional work.

Films of interest
The African Americans: Many Rivers to Cross: PBS 2013
    https://www.pbs.org/wnet/african-americans-many-rivers-to-cross/
The Doctrine of Discovery: Unmasking the Domination Code: 2014
    https://vimeo.com/ondemand/dominationcode?autoplay=1

Activity
Here's a quick quiz about the U.S.'s shared history: True or false?
1. Columbus discovered America in 1492.
2. Chinese explorers had been to North America well before the Europeans.
3. Indigenous groups in North America had engaged in economic trade with each other well before the arrival of Europeans.
4. Indigenous Peoples in North America didn't put up a fight for their land.
5. Africans did not resist being enslaved.
Critical thinking

> How did you answer the above statements? Words such as 'settled,' 'discovered,' and 'fight for' rarely convey processes that occurred over lengthy periods, nor do they do justice to others' experiences and viewpoints.
>
> If the U.S. was 'settled' by the British and other Europeans, what does this statement imply about the Indigenous Peoples of the continent who were already here and those who were forcibly brought here through enslavement? Remember the chapter on terminology. People were not 'minorities' in their own lands, they have been rendered minorities through our various histories. Additionally, how might our knowledge of extensive trade and exploration with other groups influence our view of history as well as ideas of superiority?
>
> Importantly what do these alternate views do to current conceptualizations of people and the history of *Great Turtle Island* and what we now call the U.S.? If it is true that there were established economic, governance, and political systems in place well before 1492 then Columbus clearly did not 'discover' 'America' and yet, these views have persisted for so long. Acknowledging that others had already 'discovered' and named the lands called the U.S. today does not take away from their first being *'encountered' by Europeans,* but these additional words are important. It does show regard for a more truthful version of history that accepts that Europeans were not 'the first' to know this or many other lands.

Colonization and the Impact on Health Today

Some readers may wonder why it is relevant to discuss events occurring hundreds of years ago in the context of contemporary professional practice. However, when it comes to the history of the U.S., there is evidence to suggest that colonialism remains influential in health and well-being today for everyone.

We can link many of the disease and wellness states of people today either directly or indirectly to our colonial history. For example, prior to the decimation of Native land and food resources, the diet of Native Americans was believed to have been better than that of their European counterparts. Similarly, enslavement of Africans severely disrupted food sources and diet. This is not to say that there were no health concerns previously, or that life was not challenging or without risk. Colonization, however, irrevocably disrupted the lifestyles that sustained people for thousands of years. Food sources were rendered inaccessible or destroyed.

With such forced displacement, and the establishment of reservations and plantations, came dependency on introduced foods such as lard, flour, sugar, and coffee. This dramatic change in diet and physical effort to get food led to further problems, not just in the immediate period, but also through successive generations. Flour and sugar remain staples for many Native and Black Americans. Canned, processed meats, high in sodium, known as 'spam,' have been linked to high rates of diabetes in Native communities, as is the case in other populations (Fretts et al., 2012).

Readings

There are many books and other resources relating to history and colonization and food, nutrition, diet, and health and well-being. Below is a beginning selection of readings.

Alcon, A. H., & Agyeman, J. (2011). *Cultivating food justice: Race, class, and sustainability*. Cambridge, MA: MIT Press.

Mailer, G. (2013). Decolonizing the diet: Synthesizing native American history, immunology, and nutritional science, *Journal of Evolution and Health, 1*, 1–41.

Mailer, G., & Hale, N. (2018). *Decolonizing the diet: Nutrition, immunity and the warning from early America*. New York: Anthem Press.

Mohammed, K. G. (2019). The sugar that saturates the American diet has a barbaric history as the 'white gold' that fueled slavery. The 1619 Project. https://www.hayscisd.net/cms/lib/TX02204837/Centricity/Domain/2797/Sugar%20from%20The%201619%20Project_updated.pdf

---

It is all too easy to look at historical events through contemporary lenses and respond with disbelief or judgment. The idea that anyone could arrive in an unfamiliar place today and fail to see the local inhabitants as having any rights or, worse still, to be seen as less than human, would be difficult to grasp and yet colonization still occurs. The methods might have changed in some areas from militaristic to economic strategies, but anywhere that power is asserted over others, it can be seen as colonizing practice. No doubt today's attitudes, actions, and values will also likely be subject to scrutiny in years to come. It is crucial, therefore, that the context be examined and analyzed, rather than judged.

What were the drivers of colonization? The major motivations for European communities seeking out lands beyond their own borders can be separated into three main categories:

1. religious motivation—either in seeking to convert masses or in escaping religious persecution
2. empire building—the amassing of wealth and resources, both human and material
3. overcrowding, overuse—the need for land.

As the scramble for land acquisition intensified in the late eighteenth century, it became necessary for European countries to establish some guidelines for the process. These guidelines were undoubtedly about the interests of the European superpowers and had little to do with the colonized populations. An International Court of Law was established to agree on the requirements for colonization. Three criteria by which territories could be 'legally' claimed (according to European legal systems, not the existing laws of each territory), were:

1. conquest
2. negotiation of a treaty with the original inhabitants
3. the declaration of land as belonging to no one—known as *terra nullius*.

The doctrines of discovery and notions of *terra nullius* informed much of the colonization and enslavement of people and land globally. How could anyone suggest that land was unoccupied when there was obvious evidence of people already living on the land? Well, through eighteenth-century European, Christian eyes, the Indigenous Peoples displayed no 'recognisable' signs of ownership, and, as non-Christians, they were 'heathens' and in need of 'saving.' Indigenous People's ecologically sustainable ways of living in harmony with their natural environments were in stark contrast to the European environments that were fenced and 'created'. The doctrines of discovery (domination), *terra nullius*, *and Christianity* had a profound impact on the way Indigenous and other peoples were regarded in official policies of the newly 'acquired' lands, but what relevance does it have today? We should also note that terms such as 'Christianity' and 'European' also suggest enormous diversity. Experiences and attitudes of some groups may not reflect others who may be labelled by the same terms.

Critical thinking

Consider the ongoing impact of the Doctrine of Discovery. How might this have influenced successive governments and individuals to respond to the original inhabitants? *The Doctrine of Discovery* essentially resulted in specific populations, such as Indigenous peoples on their native lands or enslaved peoples who were forcibly removed from their lands, being treated with *indifference*. Can you still see evidence of this sort of treatment today? What does it mean to treat someone with indifference? How does *indifference* relate to *mattering*?

Making it local

What evidence can you find in your local area of Indigenous-protected or significant sites? Search your local media and historical organizations. Are there any issues around sacred sites or potential tensions between particular groups? For example, look into the Black Hills as sacred land for the Lakota Sioux and the tensions relating to Mount Rushmore.

Look at the media responses to other cultural groups, both positive or negative portrayals. Can you identify any current concerns relating to

disability services, asylum seeker placements, mosques or other religious centers, or drug rehabilitation centers or other issues with a particular group?
- What knowledge do you have of the Indigenous history of where you currently live? You will need to consult a range of sources (local libraries, councils, Indigenous organizations) to find your own answers for this activity.
- Whose traditional land do you now live on?
- Whose traditional land does your workplace or university occupy?
- What Indigenous language names can you find for your local area?
- What acknowledgments or evidence can you see of an Indigenous history in your area?
- How easy or difficult was it to find the necessary information?
- What other cultural, religious, or other groups have been or currently are particularly relevant in your area? Maybe there was a significant historical event? Are there current cultural events or traditions that are still practiced that might be unique to your area?
- What, if anything, does this say about the importance given to the original inhabitants and their descendants?
- What relevance might this information have for your profession?

Past Policies

Throughout history, the government has used various policies and laws to restrict and control the lives of people and groups. These laws and policies have directly impacted basic freedoms, despite our apparent rights to life, liberty, and the pursuit of happiness. It was only in 2013 that the federal government agreed that the Defense of Marriage Act was unconstitutional, when it stated that only marriage between a man and a woman could be recognized. Prior to 2013, in most states, marriage between same-sex individuals was not legal. Many groups in the U.S. have had some form of government intrusion or management over just about every aspect of their lives since before the U.S. existed.

Reconsider the scenario of the elderly veteran who wanted to collect their hearing aid. Try to think about why their sensitivity to someone trying to control and 'manage' them might be greater than someone whose life has not been impacted in a similar way.

Key Dates and Events in History

U.S. history is unfortunately full of events, laws, and policies that negatively impacted peoples' cultures, identities, and freedoms. You may want to explore the history of events, policies, and laws for groups of interest to you. For example, search for a timeline of significant events related to LGBTQ rights. There are people still living who will remember when homosexuality was illegal in certain states and people could be jailed or lose their employment. In some cases, people were subjected to medical procedures such as castration, aversion therapies, and lobotomies to 'treat' what was deemed a mental illness until 1973 when it was declassified by the American Psychiatric Association. What is 'don't ask, don't tell' and the Stonewall Riots? You might also want to explore history as it relates to mental illness, disabilities, and religious freedoms. Think about what it might feel like to have your government tell you that you can't serve your country in the military, as has happened for transgender people. Within recent years this particular ban has been overturned, reinstated, and then overturned again.

> **Critical thinking**
> What must it be like to live through changing policy directives in one lifetime? What might it mean in terms of your day-to-day health and well-being? What might have been the rationale that underpinned each change?
> As a start, for policies affecting other groups, here are just a few things to explore: Look up the Fugitive Slave Act of 1793, the Religious Crimes Code or the Code of Indian Offenses of 1883, or the Chinese Exclusion Act of 1882.

> Look at more recent events and their aftermath and consequences and how they relate to our shared histories and our current health and well-being such as the shooting of Michael Brown and the Ferguson protests, the Charleston, South Carolina church shooting in 2015, the Black Lives Matter (BLM) protests of 2020. Do you know who Brock Turner is and his relationship to the #MeToo movement? How about Chanel Miller?

Government Responses

Various government policies have reflected, and continue to reflect, the worldview of the eras in which they were developed. By today's values, most policies were anything but benign, even though some may have arisen out of benevolent or well-meaning beliefs. How current policies will be judged by history is a matter for speculation, but the fact remains that the very policies supposedly designed to protect and assist people are undeniably implicated in the disastrous circumstances still being played out today. One of the most controversial issues has been the attempt by governments and other institutions to define individuals according to their common descent.

Definitions of Identity

Race and ethnicity definitions are governed by the 1997 Office of Management and Budget (OMB) standards on race and ethnicity. These standards guide government agencies, reports, and data collection such as that collected through the U.S. Census. Overall, a person's racial and ethnic identity is self-determined, which means that you decide which box to mark or how you describe yourself. Only since 2000 have people had the option to identify with more than one category in the U.S. Census. Five categories are required by the OMB standards as listed below (alphabetically):

American Indian or Alaska Native – A person having origins in any of the original peoples of North and South America (including Central America) and who maintains tribal affiliation or community attachment.

Asian – A person having origins in any of the original peoples of the Far East, Southeast Asia, or the Indian subcontinent including, for example, Cambodia, China, India, Japan, Korea, Malaysia, Pakistan, the Philippine Islands, Thailand, and Vietnam.

Black or African American – A person having origins in any of the Black racial groups of Africa.

Native Hawaiian or Other Pacific Islander – A person having origins in any of the original peoples of Hawaii, Guam, Samoa, or other Pacific Islands.

White – A person having origins in any of the original peoples of Europe, the Middle East, or North Africa.

Racial, ethnic, or national identity in the U.S. is not a straightforward or simplistic category, nor has it been consistent historically. We can think of identity as relating to biological descent, self-identification, and community acceptance. The element of descent relates to biology, such as your family members' identity. This could be a mother, father, grandparents, or great-grandparents, but the element is biologically determined. However, is this element a *necessary* condition for identification? Consider self-identification. For example, someone might have a great-grandparent who was Native American, but, due to a wide range of factors, perhaps this person does not 'self-identify' as Native American, despite their biological (descent) element. Is it possible for someone to self-identify as Native American without the biological element?

With the increasing popularity of DNA testing to determine ancestry, many people are now finding out possible ancestral backgrounds that they were not aware of. This may have some influence on dramatic changes in racial and ethnic identification in more recent surveys such as the census. The element of community acceptance can serve to 'authenticate' identity but think about how past policies such as the forced removal of children to boarding schools and assimilation may have compromised this community acceptance. Is a Native American who does not have tribal affiliations any less Native American? Who decides?

For American Indian or Alaska Native identity, the Bureau of Indian Affairs provides this statement:

> As a general rule, an American Indian or Alaska Native person is someone who has blood degree from and is recognized as such by a federally recognized tribe or village (as an enrolled tribal member) and/or the United States. Of course, blood quantum (the degree of American Indian or Alaska Native blood from a federally recognized tribe or village that a person possesses) is not the only means by which a person is considered to be an American Indian or Alaska Native. Other factors, such as a person's knowledge of his or her tribe's culture, history, language, religion, familial kinships, and how strongly a person identifies himself or herself as American Indian or Alaska Native, are also important. In fact, there is no single federal or tribal criterion or standard that establishes a person's identity as American Indian or Alaska Native (Bureau of Indian Affairs, n.d.).

Each tribal group makes their own determinations about who can claim tribal identity and access tribal resources. For example, the Cherokee Nation state the following for tribal registration on their website:

> The Cherokee Nation Registration Office processes Certificate of Degree of Indian Blood (CDIB), Dawes and Tribal Citizenship applications and issues CDIB, Citizenship, and Photo ID cards. The Registration office also issues Indian Preference Letters, provides verification of Tribal Citizenship, verifies eagle feather applications and provides registration services as needed.
> The basic criteria for CDIB/Cherokee Nation tribal citizenship are that an application must be submitted along with documents that directly connect a person to an enrolled lineal ancestor who is listed on the "Dawes Roll" Final Rolls of Citizens and Freedman of the Five Civilized Tribes. (Cherokee Nation, n.d.)

The Navajo Nation state the following, 'A person MUST be at least 1/4 (one quarter) Navajo to be enrolled as a member of the Navajo Nation. To determine if you are eligible for tribal membership, contact the Navajo tribe' (Navajo Nation, n.d.).

The complexities relating to identity are obvious and cannot be simplified; nevertheless, most understandings and definitions today are an improvement on the past purely biological definitions that presumed an ability to quantify 'blood'. Even so, as we see above, some tribal affiliations continue to require minimum blood degrees. This perpetuation of biological notions of identity, revealed in phrases and terms such as 'half-blood' and 'full blood' were based on extreme ethnocentrism and European notions of racial purity and impurity. Such categorizations of people were, and arguably still are, used to justify policies and practices that can be divisive and destructive.

> **Critical thinking**
> - What might be the impact of a government-imposed identity?
> - Can you come up with some examples of how 'race' or 'ethnicity' are still described in quantities, such as the Navajo Nation requirement?
> - Does it matter if someone is half or quarter Indigenous, or Irish, or Polish? And what exactly does that mean?
> - How might quantities of ethnicity or race be used in policy or by governments, tribes, or other groups to restrict or gain access to certain resources? How might the current definitions, above, be used to benefit or disadvantage certain people or groups?
> - Think about your own family heritage. Most people today have a variety of ethnicities in their background. If you had to choose, which single one would you identify with and what would be the impact on those in your family that you have to deny?
> - How does identity influence health and well-being? Does identity matter when it comes to understanding and treating health and illness?

Current Policy

Major shifts in government policy have occurred over the last few decades. Of enormous significance have been the policy developments of the current and previous federal governments. As health and human service professionals, we know that the need to validate people's pain and suffering is a key aspect of care. How might we, in the U.S., acknowledge and repair the many harms that have been inflicted on targeted groups throughout our shared history? In the most recent Presidential election of 2020, one candidate for the Democratic nomination promoted a platform of reparations and racial reconciliation and healing for the descendants of enslaved people. Let's look at some events for which there was formal acknowledgment of the harm and in some cases, reparations.

> **Activity**
> Look up some apologies in the U.S. such as the apology for the Japanese Internment Camps, the apology for the Tulsa Massacre of 1921, or the MOVE bombing of 1985 in Philadelphia (see Thompson & Slaughter, 2021).
> - What are some similarities or differences between those apologies and Obama's apology to American Indians?
> - What do these experiences tell us about the importance of having one's trauma 'witnessed and acknowledged'?
> - Why might some groups be told to 'get over it' or to just forget the past, while it would be inconceivable to expect other groups to stop engaging in recollections of harms of the past? The Holocaust, 9/11, and Pearl Harbor, for example, are often memorialized and respected as appropriate remembrances but for other groups, such as American Indians or Black Americans, seeking acknowledgment of past wrongs is often seen as problematic. What underpins these different responses?
> - Do you know anyone or have family members affected by any of these 'apologies'? What are their perspectives on the values or limitations of apologies?
> - What are the limitations of apologies? Some people criticize that apologies don't change anything. What are some advantages and disadvantages of apologies? How do reparations relate to larger processes of reconciliation in healing harms from the past?
> - What does the research tell us about the value of an apology for a wrongdoing in health care?

As health and human services professionals, there is an ethical imperative to reflect. Knowing our histories is part of reflection. When talking about history, however, there can be a disconnection between events that happened before our time and the present. In terms of the relationships between groups, history is continuous. That means historical events affecting the health of groups of people have occurred and continue to occur within the living memory of people.

> **Scenario**
> A person in their 70s is struggling to remain in their family home. Their husband wants them to consider moving into supported accommodation, but they are adamant that they do not want to go into care. They are convinced that they will be separated from their husband and made to take medication that will keep them sedated and not in control. There is no convincing the person that neither is true and their anxiety is growing.
>
> What assumptions has this scenario brought up? Who might be fearful of being separated from their life partner or forcibly treated against their will? How rational might this fear be today? How would you approach this situation? What would you need to know to allay the person's anxiety? Can you think of any historical events in the last 70 years or so that could have influenced the response?

Even a brief examination of cultural interactions since colonization will reveal the role of health and human services professionals in implementing policies that impacted negatively on people's lives. In the context of this history, consider the need to critically examine the perceived power inherent in professional roles.

Policy and Cultural Safety

Cultural safety as a philosophy requires health and human services professionals to reflect on their position in relation to those in their care. Reflection on power differences can be most obvious when the professional is from a 'majority or dominant' cultural group and the client represents a 'minority or marginalized' culture, but often, these differences are not obvious and they are very often more complicated.

Regardless, professionals are often at the forefront of policy implementation and, as such, should be mindful of the potential power this entails.

The activities associated with this chapter ask you to look at current and previous policies and developments in relation to contemporary health concerns. Reflect on the cultural safety of these policy directions and your role as an agent of policy implementation. Are 'good intentions' enough and who is it that determines what is truly in someone's 'best interest'?

Case Study: Native American Boarding Schools

The forced removal of Native American and Alaska Native children from their families is undoubtedly one of the more controversial issues within contemporary discussions of the treatment of Indigenous peoples in North America. In 1879, Richard Pratt founded the first federally funded Native American boarding school, the Carlisle Indian Industrial School, in Carlisle, Pennsylvania. Based on his philosophy to 'kill the Indian, save the man', Native American children were forced to attend these schools and not permitted to speak their Native languages or engage in any cultural practices as a way to facilitate their assimilation into Euro/American culture.

After the Department of the Interior conducted an investigation of the boarding schools in 1928, finding lack of food, overcrowding, abuse, and overall lack of care, these schools were technically all closed by the 1930s. Remnants of the boarding schools remained until the 1970s. Only since 1978 with the Indian Child Welfare Act, could Native American parents legally deny their children's placement in off-reservation schools.

For many people today, the idea that children were 'forcibly removed' is hard to comprehend. Harder still is the notion that the official policies used by government could be defined as 'genocide'. Genocide, by definition, includes the deliberate removal of children from their families with the intent to assimilate them into another culture. What do you think could be some implications for health and human services today of the Native American boarding schools? While we might look back on these events and see how these policies and practices were horrific, are there current policies and practices that are similar today, justified as being helpful? Separation of children from families in migrant detention centers and ongoing issues in child welfare and foster care show us that these concerns continue to be unresolved.

Our focus here in discussing these policies is not about applying blame or developing guilt, although some might suggest that we should. Until this history is accepted and acknowledged, it will be harder to move forward together. Many populations have experienced similarly destructive treatment. Overall, if we do not want to repeat the mistakes of the past, and if we hope for positive future outcomes, it is essential to ensure an understanding of the events and attitudes of the past that have shaped contemporary health. Unfortunately, even with such knowledge, a positive outcome is not guaranteed.

If you were to find yourself, literally overnight, subject to government intervention on the basis of some aspect of your identity alone, can you imagine the damage to any level of trust that you might have had in the healthcare and welfare systems?

Resources of interest

See the website for the Carlisle Indian School Digital Resource Center, http://carlisleindian.dickinson.edu/

This article is about the traumatic legacy of Indian boarding schools.
Pember, M. A. (2019, March 8). Death by civilization. *The Atlantic*. Accessed from: https://www.theatlantic.com/education/archive/2019/03/traumatic-legacy-indian-boarding-schools/584293/

Critical thinking
- What might be some of the legacies left by a policy such as that related to Native American Boarding Schools? Think about people you may have encountered in your professional work. Remember that many

people alive today would have been impacted by at least some policies or have family members who were.
- How might this affect their attitude and response to healthcare or human services today?

Films
Mary Frances Thompson, best known as Te Ata, was an actress and citizen of the Chickasaw Nation known for telling Native American stories. She performed as a representative of Native Americans at state dinners before President Franklin D. Roosevelt in the 1930s. *Te Ata: True story of Mary Thompson Fisher* http://www.teatamovie.com/

Dawnland is a documentary about the removal of Native American children
   https://upstanderproject.org/dawnland

Making it local
In this chapter, we began a discussion about the importance of historical events, policies, and laws on current health and well-being but have not provided all the historical and policy details—there is much more to learn. The U.S. is a big country with a very complicated history and, as we will see in coming chapters, diversity in population groups depending on where you are geographically. What can you find out about events or policies in your local area that may be relevant to health and human services? You may also want to explore in more depth the histories relating to particular groups or issues. For example, what can you learn about the history of mental illness and policies and care?

Conclusion

In this chapter, we explored various historical impacts and briefly considered how events might impact the health and well-being of people today. We explored the relevance of history as well as the role of cultural safety in understanding historical impacts on health and well-being. We further examined the impact of worldview and colonization and the implications for identity. Case studies and activities further illustrated the impacts of history on contemporary health.

Cultural safety asks us to decolonize ourselves. In order to do this, we need to recognize what it is to colonize and be colonized. It is essential for health and human services professionals to acknowledge the influences of history and experiences that can still have impacts today on all clients.

There are countless personal 'histories' of people you may work with or care for in health settings that highlight the need to be *regardful* of the power that relationships and historical influences bring to every interaction.

References

Bureau of Indian Affairs. (n.d.). *Frequently asked questions. Who is an American Indian or Alaska Native?* https://www.bia.gov/frequently-asked-questions.

Cherokee Nation. (n.d.). *Tribal registration.* https://www.cherokee.org/all-services/tribal-registration/.

DuBois, W. E. B. (1935). *Black reconstruction in America.* Oxford University Press.

Eilat-Adar, S., Zhang, Y., & Siscovick, D. S. (2012). Associations of processed meat and unprocessed red meat intake with incident diabetes: The strong heart family study. *The American Journal of Clinical Nutrition, 95*(3), 752–758. https://doi.org/10.3945/ajcn.111.029942.

Guasco, M. (2017, September 13). The misguided focus on 1619 as the beginning of slavery in the U.S. damages our understanding of American history. *Smithsonian Magazine.* https://www.smithsonianmag.com/history/

misguided-focus-1619-beginning-slavery-us-damages-our-understanding-american-history-180964873/.
National Library of Medicine. (n.d.a). *A.D. 1493: The Pope asserts rights to colonize, convert and enslave.* https://www.nlm.nih.gov/nativevoices/timeline/178.html.
National Library of Medicine. (n.d.b). *A.D. 1513: El Requirimento: Spain demands subservience.* https://www.nlm.nih.gov/nativevoices/timeline/178.html.
Newcomb, S. (2008). *Pagans in the promised land: Decoding the doctrine of Christian discovery.* Fulcrum Publishing.
Navajo Nation. (n.d.). *Frequently asked questions: How can I become an enrolled member of the Navajo Nation? How can I find my Navajo roots? (Ancestry).* https://www.navajo-nsn.gov/contact.htm.
Office of Management and Budget (OMB). (1997). *Standards on race and ethnicity.* https://www.census.gov/topics/population/race/about.html.
Smith, C. (2020, September 24). Telling the truth about slavery is not 'indoctrination'. *The Atlantic.* https://www.theatlantic.com/ideas/archive/2020/09/real-stakes-fight-over-history/616455/?fbclid=IwAR12aQFjTnK3BcmcpHp3GNLln0j96D08mql-WVZ-TYQj5wliCOYnIL-XYJM.
Thompson, P. B., & Slaughter, U. (2021). Re-Member MOVE: The anatomy of a reconciliation. *American Journal of Community Psychology, 67*, 130–141. https://doi.org/10.1002/ajcp.12478.

6

Consuming Research

In this chapter, *Consuming Research*, we discuss research from the perspective of professionals as critical consumers and provide tips and skills for assessing research quality and understanding the implications of findings for culturally safe professional practice. We discuss logic systems and worldviews as they relate to creating, developing, and interpreting research through the lens of cultural safety. Research methods and processes, including community-based participatory research, will be explored in relation to culturally safe principles. The role of unethical research in our past in contributing to distrust of health care is examined along with research ethics today.

Chapter Objectives

After completing this chapter, you should be able to:

- discuss different logic systems and worldviews that influence research
- describe some research methods commonly used in health research, including community-based participatory research

© The Author(s), under exclusive license to Springer Nature Switzerland AG 2021
P. B. Thompson and K. Taylor, *A Cultural Safety Approach to Health Psychology*, Sustainable Development Goals Series, https://doi.org/10.1007/978-3-030-76849-2_6

- discuss historical ethical issues in research and how that can contribute to current distrust in healthcare
- apply strategies for reading and assessing literature
- describe the ways professionals can be culturally safe consumers of research.

What Is Research?

What does it mean to 'research'? Research is what we do to find answers or to increase our understanding. We do it all the time. We conduct research to help us better understand an issue or a topic or maybe we have a specific question for which we are seeking an answer. Most people understand or experience research through online search engines such as Google, and certainly, this can be a good place to start. But research, in an academic sense, is substantially more than a Google search.

Consuming research—that is reading it, critiquing it, and being able to apply what is learned, is a critically important skill to have as effective, culturally safe professionals. Very few health and human service professionals will conduct research, but all should understand how to be culturally safe consumers of research.

One way to think about what we are doing with research is with the parable of 'the elephant' (Daigneault, 2013). In this parable, a group of men, who had heard about elephants, wanted to understand what an elephant was like, but were only able to examine an elephant through touch. Each undertook their own examination. Standing around the elephant, they felt what was in front of them and then compared notes. The man who touched the tail said an elephant is like a rope. One man touched the side of the elephant and proclaimed that no, it was like a wall. The man who touched the tail said the elephant was like a spear and the one who touched the trunk said an elephant was like a hose. While none of these men were wrong from their perspective, for each man, his experience of the elephant was limited and incomplete.

How can we apply the parable of the elephant to our own research or the research and information that we search for, find, interpret and apply to our lives and our work? We must constantly ask ourselves if maybe, what we think we know, or what we have learned, 'could it be wrong or incomplete?' Could there be another answer that I haven't seen? Is there another way to look at this issue that I haven't thought of? As we will see throughout this chapter, and in line with the principles of cultural safety, we always need to acknowledge that we could be wrong or there could be other equally valid viewpoints, which also means that someone else could be right or their perspective is just as acceptable as your own. Humility in research and knowledge is essential.

What has been taught in many health-related curricula in the U.S. is that ill-health and disease can be attributed to the spread of pathogens—germs. But Western medicine has not always believed in germs. Germ theory is a relatively modern-day belief that emerged out of experiments by Louis Pasteur in the 1860s (although like most things, this discovery is attributed to one individual, but others may argue its origins lay elsewhere). Yet, this theory of disease causation is so accepted today that public health and healthcare practices are based upon it.

Research in health and human services in this country has been dominated (or colonized we could say) by those with specific worldviews. Clinical control trials, medical research and quantitative research have had a privileged place in determining what is evidence. But which cultural groups do not practice some kind of research, have not developed their own bodies of knowledge or examined evidence in some way? The problem has been in the narrow, ethnocentric view that has allowed only so-called '[Western] scientific research' to dominate. Science is essential and highly valued, but it is not the domain of any single cultural group. There is an entire globe of knowledge beyond what is known as 'Western Science'.

Even within the health and psychology fields there has been competition for research grants that don't fit a narrow way of thinking. Nurses, social workers, psychologists, and others have had to push for recognition of qualitative research methodologies and to access academic journals to share findings. Qualitative research aligns more easily with Indigenous approaches, where story or narrative is valid evidence that adds more to the 'elephant' than a narrow perspective.

> **Reading**
> Smith, L. T. (2012). *Decolonizing methodologies: Research and indigenous peoples* (2nd ed.). London: Zed Books.
> This book is a valuable contribution for researchers and students to understand what it means to decolonize research practice.
> Washington, H. A. (2006). *Medical apartheid: The dark history of medical experimentation on Black Americans from colonial times to the present*. First Anchor Books.

Diunital Versus Dichotomous Logic and Worldviews

A very important part of research and understanding problems and issues is *how* we think about things, or our logical or cognitive processes, and how we view the world (i.e., our worldview). Even how we think and view the world is a part of how we ourselves are 'colonized' and requires being 'decolonized'. A *worldview* is defined as …

> A way of describing the universe and life within it, both in terms of what is and what ought to be. A given worldview is a set of beliefs that includes limiting statements and assumptions regarding what exists and what does not (either in actuality, or in principle), what objects or experiences are good or bad, and what objectives, behaviors, and relationships are desirable or undesirable. A worldview defines what can be known or done in the world, and how it can be known or done. In addition to defining what goals can be sought in life, a worldview defines what goals should be pursued. Worldviews include assumptions that may be unproven, and even unprovable, but these assumptions are superordinate, in that they provide the epistemic and ontological foundations for other beliefs within a belief system. (adapted from Koltko-Rivera, 2004, p. 2)

Researchers have long discussed variations in worldviews, philosophies, and values between groups of people such as those between

African and Euro-Americans (e.g., Bell, 1994; Carroll, 2010; Dixon, 1977; Myers, 1988). For the most part, the social sciences, and Western or Euro-American thinking in general, follow a dichotomous logic or worldview (see Table 6.1). For example, things are viewed as either good or bad, true or false, this or that, right or wrong, and even male or female and Black or White. This way of thinking is very much ingrained in Western or Euro-American culture, so much so that it can be incredibly difficult to see things in another way.

Diunital logic or worldview is another way to view things. This is an African logic system or worldview in which things can be seen as good AND bad simultaneously, or true AND false, this AND that, right AND wrong, good AND bad. The complexity and unifying aspects of

Table 6.1 A comparison of diunital and dichotomous logic or worldview with examples

Diunital (African) logic or worldview	Dichotomous (western) logic or worldview
Both/and Someone can be both a victim and perpetrator, such as with bullying and victims of bullying	*Either/or* Someone is either a bully, or a victim of bullying, but cannot be both
Union of opposites Trauma can have positive effects (such as in Post Traumatic Growth) as well as being extremely harmful (as in Post Traumatic Stress)	*Absolute answers* Trauma has absolute negative impacts and there is no point in looking for positive effects
Something can be both A and not-A at the same time Someone can be *ill* and *not ill* at the same time, such as having the flu but feeling spiritually well, or being fit and healthy but spiritually poor	*Discontinuity among things* Someone can only be sick or not sick, but not both
Perceptual oneness or unity between the observer and the observed Observation necessarily involves interactions and interpretation	*Perceptual distance or separation between the observer and the observed* Researchers can be objective in their observations of others and stand apart from the object of study
Mind and body can be one, monism or nondualism or nonduality Alcoholism can involve biology and genetics as well as spirituality, morals, and social influences	*Mind or body, Dualism* Alcoholism is a disease of the brain and genetically influenced and not a moral, social, or spiritual condition

a diunital worldview would also conceptualize the possibilities of male AND female in terms of gender identity and Black AND White in relation to race. This worldview allows for greater complexity as a way to view the world and can free us from forced dichotomous demands for strict mutually exclusive thinking.

One example of how dichotomous logic has infiltrated psychology is in the debates around nature or nurture. You will likely have been introduced to the ideas of nature and nurture in introductory psychology and maybe even in most psychology and other social science courses. Briefly, this debate concerns whether behavior is attributed to our biology and genetic makeup (nature), or our environments and upbringing (nurture). How do the diunital and dichotomous worldviews apply to this debate? As we think about health through this book, we might explore topics such as alcoholism and drug addiction, chronic illnesses, mental health and social and emotional well-being, heart conditions, and cancer and how they are understood through the lenses of nature and nurture and within the dichotomous and diunital worldviews.

As we think about the differences between diunital and dichotomous logic and worldviews, we also need to keep in mind to not make these perspectives dichotomous! While we have presented these perspectives as two very different ways to think about and view the world, the reality is that most of us may use both of these ways of thinking, depending on the situation or context. From your own experience or culture, can you identify a particular way of understanding and thinking about things that fit into these categories? Perhaps you can identify another worldview or perspective?

> **Activity**
> Looking at Table 6.1 and thinking about these two different ways of seeing the world, can you already come up with some examples that illustrate these perspectives? Look at some recent headlines or current events relevant to health and social issues. Identify how these worldviews influence how events or issues are viewed and understood. Can you reinterpret events or issues from the other perspective?

Assessing Information

Let's say we want to find something out. For example, we had a conversation the other day in our house about the race and ethnicity of people who have been shot and killed by police. The question emerged, what are the rates of death from shootings by police for different race and ethnic groups in the U.S.? Where do you look? As most people do, we started with Google.

As we looked for an answer, it was not surprising to find that question and the factors or variables we need to consider are much more complicated than originally thought. For example, who determines the race or ethnicity of these shooting victims? Who reports these incidents? Are they all reported in the same way? Does everyone have to report this information? Why or why not? What other variables or factors should we be thinking about or looking at when we try to understand what is going on? For example, does it matter if the shooting victim was carrying a firearm at the time of the shooting? Does gender matter? What about mental illness? Who is reporting the information and where did they get it from? Are they a reliable source? How would we know? What we will likely find in our search is that there is no easy answer. Indeed, we might even consider that if we think we found an answer, we very likely might be wrong, or, at least, our 'answer', is only part of the story, as with the elephant.

However, we need to start somewhere. Let's consider where we might look for information and explore some information to help us understand what we are finding.

When doing a basic internet search, you will be directed to a variety of websites. Use the CRAAP test to assess the information you find. First, is the information *Current*? Check the dates of the material you are looking at. Is the information or source *Relevant*? Who is the author of the information? Did anyone pay for or sponsor the information or the website? What are the credentials or affiliations of the author or the website? Check the domain name. If the website ends in .gov, it is a government site and .edu is an educational institution, for example.

Read the 'about' section of the website to assess who the website belongs to. Is there an author for the information you are looking for?

Can you find out any information about that author? These items all relate to the *Authority* of the source of the information. What is the *Accuracy* of the information presented? Are there sources cited and are they credible? Is the material reliable and truthful? According to whom? Was the material reviewed or refereed? This is not always easy to find out but may require further investigation. Finally, what is the *Purpose* of the information? Why is it being written or published? Are there advertisements or something being sold? Are there religious, political, or other biases evident?

Starting with a general internet search can be useful in gaining a current perspective on a topic and helping to inform your further questions and terms that you might need to know and understand before searching further. Government documents and reports can also be very useful to inform our understanding about a topic. Government departments are also required to report on their work and to make their information accessible to the public. Government departments such as the Department of Health and Human Services and the Centers for Disease Control can be good places to get an understanding of the current mainstream views on a wide range of topics.

Check the website you are looking at on a media bias chart. There are a number of media bias charts currently available that depict media and news sources and their rankings in terms of political leanings (left, right, or centrist) as well as their reliability in reporting factual information. Certainly, just because a website or news source is found to be biased in one way or the other does not mean that you need to completely discount the information. Be a 'critical consumer' of information and add it to your information to take into consideration.

> **Website**
> Use the Media Bias Chart at this website as a tool to help assess the political leanings of web-sourced information: https://www.adfontesmedia.com/

Google Scholar is a specific search engine that focuses on scholarly work. Scholarly work can include reports published through academic institutions, masters and doctoral theses, as well as peer-reviewed journal articles and other papers published in academic journals and books. After you have done an initial internet search on a topic, it's a good idea to then take your search to scholarly sources. Google Scholar can be a good first place to look for scholarly work in the field, to help narrow your search terms, and to get an idea of the broad scope of work that has been done on a topic or a research area.

Books can be good sources for detailed information about a specific topic. They can be popular or academic in nature. Edited academic books often involve researchers with a great deal of expertise and knowledge in a particular field. The authors might collate, or review, much of the research in particular fields or subject areas. A limitation of books is that they are typically not peer-reviewed, though this does not necessarily reduce the value of the material.

Theses and dissertations can be useful sources for cutting edge thinking about a topic and can provide a wide range of sources relevant to a particular field. Academic publications often emerge from theses and dissertations.

Scholarly journal articles or academic publications might include systematic reviews, research reports, opinions, rapid reports, and first-person accounts. Peer-reviewed journal articles often have strict word limits requiring researchers to summarize their work very concisely. These publications undergo a review process where other experts in the field anonymously scrutinize the work. This process can be time-consuming, sometimes taking years to complete. It is not unusual for a research project to be published five years or more after the study was conducted.

Gray literature is other information that can be very useful but not published in the other forms mentioned. This literature might include reports from non-profit organizations, educational institutions, or other agencies who work closely with communities but do not have the capacity or resources (or even interest) to elevate information to a form such as an academic publication or book.

> **Reading**
> Nicholas, G. (2018). When scientists 'discover' what Indigenous people have known for centuries: When it supports their claims, Western scientists value what Traditional Knowledge has to offer. If not, they dismiss it. *Smithsonian Magazine*. https://www.smithsonianmag.com/science-nature/why-science-takes-so-long-catch-up-traditional-knowledge-180968216/

Research Methods

Research methods are what we do to collect information or data. These are the ways that we set out to test our ideas, theories, or assumptions about the world, events, behaviors, and such. Overall, research in the social and health sciences involves being a good observer, whether that involves observing people and their behaviors or the ways that they interact, or observing results or research findings through numbers, graphs, figures, or patterns in conversations. Our methods might include interviews, sending out a survey, or collecting a variety of biological information, such as blood tests, urine samples, blood pressure, or body weight. The kinds of information we collect can be in the form of numbers (often called quantitative data) or words (qualitative data). We might describe our observations in a variety of ways to show how they relate to one another or to our ideas.

Randomized Controlled Trials

We often find in health and social sciences that the randomized controlled trial is viewed as the 'gold standard' of research methods and is the ultimate method to determine causality. Causality is the idea or principle that everything has a cause and that, through rigorous research methods, we can determine cause and effect. This information constitutes much of what is deemed 'evidence' and, in theory, guides the work that health and human services professionals do. 'Evidence-based practice' is applying 'scientific evidence' to our work and to the decisions we make. Some have gone so far as to say that *only* work or practice that has been proven or supported by rigorous, scientific evidence should be implemented. Read the following abstract from researchers skeptical of the strict requirement for 'evidence' based wholly on randomized controlled trials:

> Objectives: To determine whether parachutes are effective in preventing major trauma related to gravitational challenge.
> Design: Systematic review of randomised controlled trials.
> Data sources: Medline, Web of Science, Embase, and the Cochrane Library databases; appropriate internet sites and citation lists.
> Study selection: Studies showing the effects of using a parachute during free fall.
> Main outcome measure: Death or major trauma, defined as an injury severity score > 15.
> Results: We were unable to identify any randomised controlled trials of parachute intervention.
> Conclusions: As with many interventions intended to prevent ill health, the effectiveness of parachutes has not been subjected to rigorous evaluation by using randomised controlled trials. Advocates of evidence-based medicine have criticised the adoption of interventions evaluated by using only observational data. We think that everyone might benefit if the most radical protagonists of evidence-based medicine organised and participated in a double blind, randomised, placebo controlled, crossover trial of the parachute. (Smith & Pell, 2003)

Overall, there are many methods that can be used in research to help us better understand our clients, their situations, and how we can best serve them. Some methods will be more successful in some contexts and not successful in other contexts. And sometimes, like in the parachute example, we just need to think carefully and critically and use our experiences, knowledge, and communication with our clients to determine what might be the best course of action.

Ethics and Research

Health services and medical care are overwhelmingly viewed or believed to be part of the solution to health problems and concerns, and most of the time this is true. Indeed, medical professionals take the Hippocratic Oath to 'do no harm'. But what about when health care is the problem? Researchers from Johns Hopkins University found that medical errors are the third leading cause of death in the U.S., with about 250,000 deaths from medical errors occurring every year (Makary & Daniel, 2016). Certainly, mistakes are bound to happen, but we are also justified in being cautious about the care we receive and perhaps seeking a second opinion. In addition to general mistakes that can happen in the course of our health care, there are unfortunately numerous examples of harm inflicted through medical care and unethical research practices.

The Tuskegee Study of Untreated Syphilis in the Negro Male was a study conducted between 1932 and 1972 in Alabama. This is probably the most well-known study of medical racism and unethical research practices in the U.S., but unfortunately, it is not the only case. In the Tuskegee study, treatment was withheld from around 200 participants. While there were no proven treatments for syphilis when the study began, the use of penicillin to treat syphilis was the standard treatment in 1947.

As part of a blinding control procedure, the men in the study who were in the control group were told that they were being treated when they were not. Blinding in a research study means that the research participants do not know what treatment condition they are in. When a study has an experimental group and a control group, the control group typically does not receive the treatment but may receive a placebo, or a substance that does not have an effect. Not only did the research participants continue to get sick and even die, but also had infected others in the community.

Researchers did not tell the men in the study the true title of the study or the nature of their illness (they were only told that they had 'bad blood'). Despite concerns being raised about the ethics of the study as early as 1968, it wasn't until 1972 when news articles condemned the study and it was eventually ended. Hearings and a class-action lawsuit began in 1973 and in 1997 President Clinton apologized to study participants and their families.

As a health or human services professional, it is important to understand the history and contemporary possibilities for mistakes and unethical practices. It is also important to understand that there are guidelines and codes for the conduct of research to help prevent problematic practices from occurring. For example, the Nuremberg Code of 1947 required that research participants voluntarily consent to participate in research. The Nuremberg Code, a set of ten ethical principles for research, resulted from the trials following WWII of doctors who had conducted cruel medical experiments in concentration camps in Nazi Germany. The following are the ten principles:

1. Voluntary, informed consent is essential
2. The results of any experiment must be for the greater good of society and not random or unnecessary
3. Human experiments should be based on previous animal experimentation
4. Experiments should be conducted in a way that avoids physical and mental suffering and injury
5. No experiments should be conducted if it is believed to cause death or disability
6. The risks should never exceed the benefits of the research
7. Adequate facilities should be used to protect subjects from injury, disability, or death
8. Experiments should be conducted only by scientifically qualified persons
9. Subjects should be able to end their participation at any time
10. The scientist in charge must be prepared to terminate the experiment when injury, disability, or death is likely to occur.

Other recommended sources

> Declaration of Helsinki (2000), originally World Medical Association in 1964. These are principles that are directed toward physicians, but are relevant to medical research
> https://www.wma.net/policies-post/wma-declaration-of-helsinki-ethical-principles-for-medical-research-involving-human-subjects/
> Belmont Report (1979)
> https://www.hhs.gov/ohrp/regulations-and-policy/belmont-report/read-the-belmont-report/index.html
> CIOMS (2002): Council for International Organizations of Medical Sciences: International Ethical Guidelines for Biomedical Research Involving Human Subjects 2016: International Ethical Guidelines for Health-Related Research Involving Humans
> https://cioms.ch/wp-content/uploads/2017/01/WEB-CIOMS-EthicalGuidelines.pdf
> National Institutes of Health: Patient Recruitment: Ethics in Clinical Research: Ethical Guidelines https://clinicalcenter.nih.gov/recruit/ethics.html
> National Institutes of Health: Guiding Principles for Ethical Research: https://www.nih.gov/health-information/nih-clinical-research-trials-you/guiding-principles-ethical-research

Community-Based Participatory Research

Community-based participatory research and other similar research approaches such as participatory action research are research processes that have been shown to address some of the concerns with other research practices. Hartwig et al. (2006) suggest community-based participatory research as a method can be useful particularly because traditional research has failed to solve complex health disparities and many communities and groups are burned out. Also, research design and results can be improved when community members are actively involved in all stages of the research process. Research findings can be applied more effectively when communities are involved as equal partners. Overall, when relationships are an integral part of the entire research process, research and health outcomes are improved.

Community-based participatory research provides a research process that fits well with the principles of cultural safety. When community members are active and equal partners throughout the research process, this can be decolonizing and address power imbalances. Communication throughout the research process, in the determination of the need for research, the development of the research protocols and methods, the interpretation of findings, and finally, the application of those findings, improves the quality of the research and benefits all who are involved.

Special Topic: Culture and Population Migration: Female Circumcision

In this next section, we will look at a special topic and see how we can apply a culturally safe, critical analysis. Many people are familiar with the practice of male circumcision, but most will not have heard that there is also a tradition of female circumcision in many countries around the world. Greater awareness of female circumcision emerged when practicing communities migrated to western countries and western health professionals found themselves ill-equipped and ill-informed. We can learn a lot about culturally safe (and unsafe) healthcare and human services practices by exploring this particular practice and how, when very different cultural practices come together through population migration patterns, misunderstandings can lead to quick decisions with severe consequences for communities. We will see how we can apply a decolonizing and culturally safe lens through which to interpret research and policy. The practice of female circumcision also provides us with a good example for understanding diunital and dichotomous logic.

As a start to our discussion of this cultural practice, let's first look at the terms that are used to describe it. The World Health Organization calls the practice 'Female Genital Mutilation' (FGM), as does most mainstream media. But if we were to ask women in communities who engage in this practice, we would find a range of other labels or descriptions such as cutting, sunna, or circumcision. Understandably, many find the label Female Genital Mutilation offensive and hypocritical. As we think about cultural safety, imagine your own cultural traditional practice being given the label of 'mutilation'. A range of emotions, images, and potential misunderstandings have been created before we even start the conversation.

Remember earlier we talked about cultural safety as involving a cycle of awareness, sensitivity, and safety? Think about how someone who is new to learning about this cultural practice, and therefore developing an awareness, may be biased when the topic itself is initially presented as 'mutilation'. To become aware of a cultural practice, it is important to be introduced to the topic without layers of stigma, bias, and discrimination that will now need to be unpacked and destigmatized. In this spirit, let's take a look at some of the basics of this practice and consider how we might move toward cultural safety.

The WHO (2020) recognizes four categories of the practice, aptly called Type I, Type II, Type III, and Type IV. Type I, also sometimes called Sunna in Muslim practicing communities, is the 'partial or total removal of the clitoral glans (the external and visible part of the clitoris, which is a sensitive part of the female genitals), and/or the prepuce/clitoral hood (the fold of skin surrounding the clitoral glans)'. Type III, also called infibulation or pharaonic circumcision, has attracted the most attention because of the severity of the practice. It is defined by the WHO as 'the narrowing of the vaginal opening through the creation of a covering seal. The seal is formed by cutting and repositioning the labia minora, or labia majora, sometimes through stitching, with or without removal of the clitoral prepuce/clitoral hood and glans (Type I)'.

Given the definitions of Type I and Type III circumcisions, do you think that health effects of these two very different procedures might also be very different? Can you think of any practices or traditions in Western cultures that may be similar to these procedures? While a very different body part (or is it?), some have compared the practice to various body piercing practices, which in some communities is done with newborns or very young children.

The practices of female circumcision vary widely both within and between communities and families. The age of circumcision ranges from girls who are very young, as young as two (although this is unusual), and into adulthood. Female circumcision is practiced by a wide range of religious groups including Christians, Muslims, Jewish, and Animists. Female circumcisions are more common in African, Middle Eastern, and Asian countries, but due to migration, including forced migration, the practice is now seen globally. Circumcision may be performed under medical conditions or by a midwife or woman who has been trained or selected by the community. When circumcision is performed by untrained people and in unsanitary conditions, unsurprisingly, infections and problems can arise. Additionally, childbirth can be complicated for women who are infibulated especially when they are being treated by healthcare professionals unfamiliar with the practice and with deinfibulation procedures. It is these cases, particularly with Type III circumcision, when infections, botched procedures, and other complications can arise, as well as ethnocentrism (applying one's own cultural perspectives onto another culture or practice), that have attracted so much attention. While some researchers and professionals have argued that medicalization of the practice would reduce harm and problems, the WHO is opposed to medicalization.

Let's explore how diunital and dichotomous logic apply to the case of female circumcision. Calling the practice Female Genital Mutilation creates a dichotomous perspective in that the practice has been put into a box of 'bad' and any attempts to talk about the practice in a less-stigmatized way may lead to being labelled as condoning the practice and potentially in support of child abuse and violence against women. The naming of the practice, in and of itself, potentially prevents conversations and inhibits research, understanding and community engagement. For example, the WHO states that there are no benefits to the practice. But could there be? For example, we know that male circumcision can have health benefits for both males and their female partners (Eisenberg et al., 2018). We can't even begin to explore the possibilities with female circumcision due to the heated context surrounding the practice. How does this relate to diunital and dichotomous logic? Thinking about the different models of health that we explored earlier, what might be some of the questions we could ask regarding 'benefits' of a cultural practice? Are benefits only understood in terms of biology? Or should we consider social and relational, religious or spiritual, emotional, or any other outcomes?

Within the framework of cultural safety, it is important to look at history and how it is related and to look at oneself critically. For female circumcision, with the outrage that we see from U.S. academics, advocacy groups, and health professionals, one would think that no one in the U.S. ever engaged in any sort of manipulation of the female genitalia. However, there is a long history and current practices that often fail to be acknowledged.

Rodriguez (2014) explores the history of female circumcision and clitorectomy in the U.S., showing an extensive history as well as an increase in current 'female genital cosmetic surgeries'. For example, 'following liposuction, breast augmentation and rhinoplasty, labiaplasty was reported to be the fourth most common cosmetic surgical procedure according to U.S. statistics in 2013, rising by 44% in 2013 alone' (Simonis et al., 2016). Labiaplasty, vulvoplasty, and other female genital cosmetic surgeries include trimming of the labia minora and less commonly labia majora, hymenoplasty, vaginal reconstruction, mons pubis liposuction, vaginal 'rejuvenation' or laser 'rejuvenation', G-spot augmentation, and Orgasm-shot. Revisit the description of Type III 'FGM'. Do you see any similarities?

If we broaden our scope, we might also look at other body modification practices such as tattooing, piercing, and scarification and ask ourselves if the extreme response to female genital circumcisions is warranted. Indeed, even Healthline, a well-known source for medical and health information, has a special section on their website for 'clitoris piercing'. Moulton and Jernigan (2017) found that women are increasingly having genital piercings and suggest an increase in complications.

Consider other practices such as abortion that continue to be a contentious topic in the U.S. as it relates to legality and the implications of that for health care and outcomes. Making abortion illegal potentially forces the practice underground, and thereby with no protections to prevent unhealthy and unsafe procedures. Women have historically engaged in a wide range of practices when faced with an unwanted or forced pregnancy that have led to complications and even death. While it has taken decades to legalize safe abortions under medical conditions in the U.S., it continues to be a contentious and politically heated topic. Despite the politics, the benefits of abortions in medical settings as opposed to non-medical settings are unquestionable.

But it seems there is no possibility of medicalization and harm minimization for female circumcision, at least for African and other women who practice this culturally. Thirty-nine states have laws against the practice of 'FGM' and in 2021, the STOP FGM Act of 2020 was signed into law. This law gives federal authorities the power to prosecute those who carry out or conspire to carry out FGM, as well as increasing the maximum prison sentence from five to ten years. It also requires government agencies to report to Congress about the estimated number of females who are at risk of or have had FGM, and on efforts to prevent FGM (Stop FGM Act of 2020). This may be understandable to protect those under the age of consent for medical procedures, but why is the same protection not given to young boys in response to the still common practice of circumcision? Just to be clear, we are not advocating for these practices. We are asking professionals who may encounter cultural practices at odds with their own worldview, to critically analyze your responses, assumptions, and judgments in your professional practice. This includes asking hard and unpopular questions with curiosity and a desire to understand and learn.

The Somali community has attracted a lot of attention in relation to the practice because many of the women have experienced the Type III circumcision and it is still practiced although there is evidence that this is changing (Guerin et al., 2006). The Somali diaspora (or the dispersion of a people) grew dramatically since the 1990s with the Somali Civil War. Somali people had long been travelers as merchants and perhaps had been coming to North America since the 1850s. Through the United Nations High Commissioner for Refugees program, many Somali were relocated to the U.S., New Zealand, Australia, Canada, and throughout Europe. There are currently around 150,000 Somali living in the U.S. (Connor & Krogstad, 2016).

Given what we have learned in this brief review of female circumcision, how might women in a community like the Somali community be affected by legislation against the practice and the ways in which the practice is framed or discussed?

> **Critical thinking**
> Are genital cosmetic surgeries or genital piercings considered FGM? If they are not, why not? And, if they are not, then is the FGM law inherently racist?
> What do you do when your own values and beliefs are in conflict with those of your clients? How do you navigate your professional practice?
> How do these words, such as 'mutilated' or 'cosmetic surgery' reflect or influence your worldview?

> **Reading**
> Below is an excellent review that applies cultural safety to the healthcare experiences of those who have experienced female circumcision.
> Evans, C., Tweheyo, R., McGarry, J., et al. (2019). Seeking culturally safe care: A qualitative systematic review of the healthcare experiences of women and girls who have undergone female genital mutilation/cutting. *BMJ Open, 9,* e027452. https://doi.org/10.1136/bmjopen-2018-027452.

> **Making it local**
> Using Google Scholar, type in key words for your state or local community, including the words **health psychology** or **health services**. Find an article that relates to your area or region. Ideally, look at research from the last five years for this activity. For example, a search including the key terms above and Oklahoma brought up a number of articles including:
> Currin, J. M, Hubach, R., Crethar, H., Hammer, T. R., Lee, H., & Larson, M. (2018). Barriers to accessing mental healthcare for gay and

> bisexual men living in Oklahoma. *Sexuality Research and Social Policy, 15,* 483–496.
>
> The same search using Hawaii, elicited this article:
>
> Lim, E., Gandhi, K., Siriwardhana, C., Davis, J., & Chen, J. J. (2019). Racial and ethnic differences in mental health service utilization among the Hawaii medicaid population. *Journal of Mental Health, 28*(5), 536–545. https://doi.org/10.1080/09638237.2018.1521917
>
> Sometimes the articles are restricted for purchase, but often they are free access. Read the abstract to determine if this would be a useful article to learn more about what research has been conducted in your local area. Do these research studies reflect any cultural safety principles in their processes? If not, why not? What would need to happen to make them culturally safe?

Conclusion

Research is a valuable tool for understanding the world, but as with the perspectives of those investigating the elephant by feel only, it can be limited and unsafe if it only takes into consideration a narrow perspective. Research that contributes to greater understanding will be culturally safe, decolonized in methods and methodology, ethical, and not privilege certain worldviews over others.

References

Bell, Y. R. (1994). A culturally sensitive analysis of black learning style. *Journal of Black Psychology, 20*(1), 47–61. https://doi.org/10.1177/00957984940 2001005.

Carroll, K. K. (2010). A genealogical review of the worldview framework in African-centered psychology. *The Journal of Pan African Studies, 3*(8), 109–134.

Connor, P., & Krogstad, J. M. (2016, June 1). *5 facts about the global Somali diaspora*. Pew Research Centre. https://www.pewresearch.org/facttank/2016/06/01/5-facts-about-the-global-somali-diaspora/.

Daigneault, P.M. (2013). The blind men and the elephant: A metaphor to illuminate the role of researchers and reviewers in social science. *Methodological Innovations Online, 8*(2), 82–89. https://doi.org/10.4256/mio.2013.015.

Dixon, V. J. (1977). African-oriented and Euro-American-oriented world views: Research methodologies and economics. *The Review of Black Political Economy, 7*, 119–156.

Eisenberg, M. L., Galusha, D., Kennedy, W. A., & Cullen, M. R. (2018). The relationship between neonatal circumcision, urinary tract infection, and health. *The World Journal of Men's Health, 36*(3), 176–182. https://doi.org/10.5534/wjmh.180006.

Guerin, P. B., Allotey, P., Hussein Elmi, F., & Baho, S. (2006). Advocacy as a means to an end: Assisting refugee women to take control of their reproductive health needs. *Women Health, 43*(4), 7–25. https://doi.org/10.1300/J013v43n04_02. PMID: 17135086.

Hartwig, K., Calleson, D., & Williams, M. (2006). Unit 1: Community-based participatory research: Getting grounded. In: The Examining Community-Institutional Partnerships for Prevention Research Group. *Developing and Sustaining Community-Based Participatory Research Partnerships: A Skill-Building Curriculum*. www.cbprcurriculum.info.

Koltko-Rivera, M. E. (2004). The psychology of worldviews. *Review of General Psychology, 8*(1), 3–58.

Kelley, A., Belcourt-Dittloff, A., Belcourt, C., & Belcourt, G. (2013, December). Research ethics and Indigenous communities. *American Journal of Public Health, 103*(12), 2146–2152. https://doi.org/10.2105/AJPH.2013.301522. https://www.ncbi.nlm.nih.gov/pmc/articles/PMC3828983/.

Makary, M. A., & Daniel, M. (2016). Medical error—The third leading cause of death in the U.S. *British Medical Journal, 353*, i2139. https://doi.org/10.1136/bmj.i2139.

Moulton, L. J., & Jernigan, A. M. (2017). Management of retained genital piercings: A case report and review. *Case Reports in Obstetrics and Gynecology*, 2402145. https://doi.org/10.1155/2017/2402145.

Myers, L. (1988). *Understanding an Afrocentric worldview: Introduction to an optimal psychology*. Kendall/Hunt.

Rich, K., & Breunig, M. (2020). Cultural safety: A lens to consider leisure provision in cross-cultural contexts. *Managing Sport and Leisure*. https://doi.

org/10.1080/23750472.2020.1800506. https://www.tandfonline.com/doi/abs/10.1080/23750472.2020.1800506.

Rodriguez, S. B. (2014). *Female circumcision and clitoridectomy in the United States: A history of a medical treatment*. University of Rochester Press.

Simonis, M., Manocha, R., & Ong, J. J. (2016). Female genital cosmetic surgery: A cross-sectional survey exploring knowledge, attitude and practice of general practitioners. *BMJ Open, 6*(9), e013010. https://doi.org/10.1136/bmjopen-2016-013010.

Smith, G. C. S., & Pell, J. P. (2003). Parachute use to prevent death and major trauma related to gravitational challenge: Systematic review of randomised controlled trials. *British Medical Journal, 327*, 1459. https://doi.org/10.1136/bmj.327.7429.1459.

Stop FGM Act of 2020. H. R. 6100. 116th Congress (2019–2020). Public Law No. 116-309. https://www.congress.gov/bill/116th-congress/house-bill/6100/text.

WHO. (2020). *Female genital mutilation fact sheet*. https://www.who.int/news-room/fact-sheets/detail/female-genital-mutilation.

7

Determinants of Health

Determinants of Health explores the influences on health beyond an individual's biological or behavioral health. These influences include education, poverty, employment, and housing. Importantly, all of these influences are also determined by politics, racism, and discrimination. Readers will be encouraged to reflect on their own cultures and identities and the potential impact on others; to identify examples of systemic bias, institutional and individual racism and discrimination; and to analyze and discuss determinants of health.

Chapter Objectives

After completing this chapter, you should be able to:

- identify the determinants of health from a broader perspective than biomedical
- reflect on your own cultures and identities and their potential impact on others

- identify examples of systemic bias, institutional and individual racism and discrimination
- analyze and discuss concepts of racism and discrimination and their impact on professional care.

Determinants of Health Explained

Ultimately, our goal for culturally safe health care and systems is health equity. To build our awareness, our sensitivity, and the safety of our practices and systems, an understanding of all of the factors that impact health and well-being is critical.

Health is determined by much more than biological influences as we have already noted in previous chapters. In fact, the health and well-being of individuals has less to do with an individual's diet and exercise and more to do with experiences of health care and social contexts including families and communities and the built environments in which we live.

There is a substantial body of literature relating to the 'determinants of health'. Most often these 'determinants' are described as the 'social determinants of health' to distinguish them from the purely biological contributors to health. The 'social' determinants are a way to explain the broader causal factors that lead to ill-health. These social determinants of health include factors such as access to education, housing, income, and employment and political factors (Dawes, 2020). These factors are collectively referred to as *socioeconomic status*, or SES, which is a *determinant* of health as it is critically important in understanding the current state of health. Particular groups of people are more likely to experience poor socioeconomic conditions compared to dominant or privileged groups.

However, keep in mind that low or poor socioeconomic conditions are a value judgment made through the lens of capitalism and wealth, in an economic sense, and may not necessarily reflect the diversity of notions of 'wealth'. Dominant culture perspective often defines what these determinants are, how they are measured and interpreted, and how they are judged and understood. Education for example, often implies Western education, with particular judgments of benchmarks, such as completion of high school or higher education. Indeed, we refer to education past high school as 'higher', as if it is 'superior' or 'better' than other forms of education such as in the trades or arts or small businesses or even life experiences. Housing and employment are also defined by Western and capitalist ideas and values and are the metric for determining and judging health and well-being such as home ownership or whether someone is employed part-time, full-time, or self-employed.

Social determinants, however, are strongly linked to health outcomes, but not exclusively and not always for people who may conceive of an entirely different set of determinants of health. For example, Reid and Taylor (2011) discuss the importance of maintaining Indigenous core values to engage in the world. An individual who maintains their functioning through the key values of respect, reciprocity, and relationships, for example, may be considered healthy, even in the absence of employment, education, or shelter as conceptualized from a Western perspective. Determinants of health from other perspectives and worldviews need to be included in health and academic discourses. Let's now take a closer look at what has been described as the social determinants of health.

Readings

Dawes, D. E. (2020). *The political determinants of health.* Baltimore: Johns Hopkins University Press.

Marmot, M. (2015). *The health gap: The challenge of an unequal world.* Bloomsbury.

In 2005, the World Health Organization established the Commission on the Social Determinants of Health, which included a global network of researchers, policymakers, and civil society organizations (WHO, 2008). The Commission on the Social Determinants of Health focused on nine broad areas that contain themes. These themes are employment conditions, social exclusion, priority public health conditions, women and gender equity, early child development, globalization, health systems, measurement and evidence, and urbanization.

The Rio Political Declaration on the Social Determinants of Health was adopted in October 2011 at the World Conference of the Social Determinants of Health in Rio de Janeiro. This declaration includes five priority areas: enhancing health policies and decision-making, widening participation in policymaking and implementation, improving health care and services, strengthening international cooperation, and monitoring impact and progress (WHO, 2011).

The CDC describes the social determinants of health as the conditions in the places where people live, learn, work, and play that affect a wide range of health risks and outcomes (CDC, n.d.). *Healthy People 2030* outlines five key areas of the social determinants of health including healthcare access and quality, education access and quality, social and community context, economic stability and neighborhood, and built environment. These circumstances are shaped by the distribution of money, power, and resources at global, national, and local levels. Health outcomes are influenced by economic policies and systems, development agendas, social norms, social policies, and political systems (WHO, n.d.).

Health inequities, or the unfair and avoidable differences in health status that we see both within and between countries, are influenced by the social determinants of health. These determinants include income, education, employment and job security, food insecurity, the conditions of working life, housing, amenities and environmental conditions, social support and inclusion, structural conflicts, early child development and access to quality and affordable health care.

If we consider colonization and the history of policies that impacted many groups in the U.S., we might come up with a description of the social conditions that many people are likely to experience. For example, we might say that these groups are more likely to:

- die younger
- live with higher levels of chronic illness
- be under-educated, un- or under-employed, and economically disadvantaged
- be or have been imprisoned
- live in overcrowded or inadequate housing.

These experiences and social contexts have been documented and reported for many years. However, remember that although statistically a greater proportion of people from certain groups are likely to experience lower social and economic status, this does not mean it is true for everyone in those groups. We need to be aware of the potential for further biases and stereotypes to develop when we learn about various inequalities. Additionally, at least some statistics and data analysis are based on Western ideals and judgments that may not provide a balanced perspective. Even considering these issues, statistically there are differences between groups that certainly warrant attention or further investigation.

Culture and Identity as Determinants of Health and Well-Being

We have discussed culture and identity extensively already throughout this book. But how can someone's culture or identity *determine* their health and well-being? 'Culture dictates the language used to define issues, the identification of problems, the framing of those problems, the manner in which solutions are sought, and the methods for defining and measuring success' (Knibb-Lamouche, 2012). Culture, or identity, are the intersecting aspects of who you are, as a person, and the overlapping of these aspects with the people around you. This might include your relationships, your communication, how you see yourself, and how you relate to the world around you.

Culture or identity as a determinant of health and well-being relates to the 'fit' between you and all the places and spaces you engage with as you live your life. Maya Angelou (1986) wrote that 'the ache for home lives in all of us, the safe place where we can go as we are and not be questioned'. Some people have lots of 'safe places', but for others, these 'safe places' are few and far between. Frequent exposure to 'unsafe places' or places where your identity or culture are questioned, challenged, or, demeaned, can result in a range of health issues such as chronic physical or what are often described as 'mental illnesses'.

It's not difficult to understand then why it is so essential to ensure the cultural safety of people accessing health and human services. There is significant evidence to support what many have already known: that cultural maintenance and vitality adds to resilience. Our nation's history, however, is one of assault and disruption to cultures and identities, leaving people vulnerable and harmed.

How people feel in society—their sense of belonging, which is somewhat influenced by how they are treated by others—is an important element in determining the health of individuals, their families, and communities. When someone treats another person in a way that diminishes, disempowers, or demeans them then this treatment may be racist or discriminating, but most people are not willing to admit that their actions may be such. Many people in the U.S. experience racism and discrimination, which evidence shows has a damaging impact on health and well-being.

The chapter on History highlights the disturbing situation of government 'sanctioned' discrimination against various groups throughout our history and this discrimination continues, albeit, often more subtly. Although cultural safety asks us to treat people 'regardful' of their differences, *when different treatment is imposed or when it results in poorer outcomes, then that treatment is racist or discriminatory.*

Education

A major social determinant of health is an individual's educational levels. How do we define 'education'? Descriptions of people as 'uneducated' or 'illiterate' fail to acknowledge the social and cultural education that is so much a part of many societies. Discussions and assessments of 'education' almost exclusively relate to education as a formalized, Western, school education. In the following discussion, we will refer to education using this definition and we will consider the implications for health in that context.

Research indicates that every year of formal school education undertaken by a young woman can dramatically influence the health outcomes for her entire family. The links between health and education are increasingly clear. Government policies that allowed for the exclusion or segregation of children based on race and ethnicity and gender, ensured educational disadvantage. There may be some readers of this book who are first in their families to attend formal education after high school. What might some of the barriers have been for others in your family in the past?

Just as with health, problems of access and acceptability in education continue to negatively impact educational levels. The cycle goes on, as we see in Fig. 7.1.

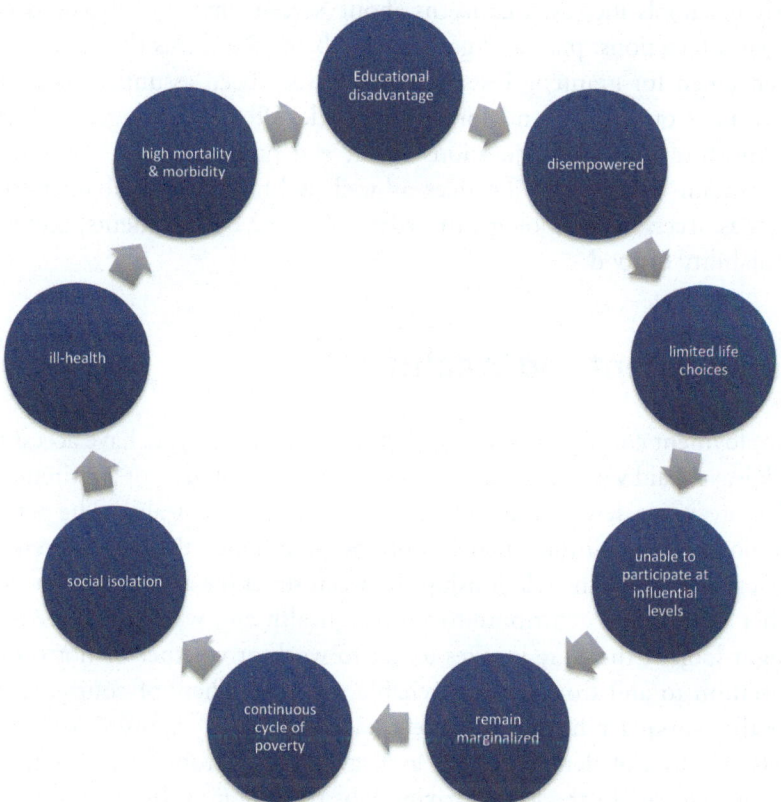

Fig. 7.1 Impact of educational disadvantage (Taylor & Thompson-Guerin, 2019)

Formal, Western education alone is clearly only one part of a still elusive solution. Much of the focus often seems to be on what people should or shouldn't do to improve their health. However, consider this: what 'education' might be required for people to shift from stigmatizing specific health service users to understanding and reinforcing the efforts people do make for their health?

The 2020 COVID-19 pandemic drastically changed the education environment, challenging many practices that had been normalized and inflexible for so long. Suddenly, home-schooling parents previously chided were highly sought-out experts. Long hours every day attending virtual schools increased concerns about 'screen time' and the need for social interactions, play, and general well-being, concerns that often had been taken for granted. Tests that had always been assumed necessary were now optional or no longer required. All these changes brought to the fore important questions about the purpose, value, and need for certain educational practices as well as broader societal inequities such as access to technology, the safety of home environments, and the availability of food.

Employment and Wealth

Employment conditions such as whether or not employees have access to sick leave, paid vacations, parental leave, health insurance, or a retirement plan are just a few of the factors that can influence health. The actual employment conditions such as working long hours, the stressfulness of the environment, the relationships between superiors and co-workers are other factors that contribute to people's health and well-being. We also might look at the time it takes to get to work or whether or not transportation to and from work is reliable and safe. Then, of course, there are the workplace health and safety hazards such as exposure to chemicals or physical demands such as heavy lifting. Ironically, it is those people who are in the lowest paying jobs that are most likely to get sick or injured who are most in need of health insurance and health care. Minimum wage in the U.S. has not kept up with the increasing costs of housing, food, clothing, and other basic necessities.

And what about unemployment? It would not be hard to imagine the challenges of losing a job and income on health. This book is not presenting figures but we encourage readers to conduct a search for national, state, and local figures. The rates of unemployment in some areas are dire and the ongoing impact means that there are sectors of the community who live in economically impoverished conditions, right here in the U.S., an economically wealthy nation. This level of disadvantage within a country can often go unnoticed or hidden as people struggle to maintain a veneer of 'normalcy'. When money is tight, the first things to let go of are often the very things that maintain health. When stress increases, the coinciding pattern of spending can be on things like tobacco, alcohol, or drugs. This does not mean that tobacco and substance abuse is always associated with the unemployed and low-income populations, but these can be symptoms of an individual or group in crisis.

Income or wealth are other contributors to health and well-being. It is not just the amount of money or wealth that someone has, although if you have 'enough' money, certainly, stressors related to being able to afford the basic necessities are eliminated. Patterns of wealth and poverty and the equitable distribution of resources also matter. Inequities in the distribution of wealth have been shown to be highly correlated with a range of health and social outcomes (Marmot, 2015).

Disparities in income, between people in the same jobs, is yet another concern that negatively impacts on health and well-being. Imagine finding out that a co-worker earns more than you—for the same job and the same qualifications. The American *myth of meritocracy* will have you believe that if you just work harder you will get there too, or that people who are very economically wealthy have 'earned' it. But someone who earns $500,000 per year does not 'work' 10 times harder, nor are they 10× 'smarter' than someone who earns $50,000.

Wealth in the U.S. is generally understood as material possessions, money, and resources or 'being rich'. But from a cultural safety perspective, remember that not everyone has the same understandings or values regarding 'wealth'. One indicator of social status, or wealth, for many people is demonstrated by questions about family and children. Those without family, or with no children of their own, can be met with expressions of pity, as these are the hallmarks of 'wealth' in some settings, rather than material 'wealth'. Rich cultural practices and strong cultural identities are essential and protective to health and social and emotional well-being.

Housing, Overcrowding, and Houselessness

Housing has long been recognized as a critical factor contributing to health and well-being. The quality of the house that people occupy, housing tenure (whether you own your house or rent), and the neighborhood characteristics (for example, whether you have spaces or places for exercise or the safety of the neighborhood), all contribute to people's health.

The Flint Water Crisis drew attention across the country to issues of water quality, particularly in urban areas with old homes and lead pipes. Poor water quality can be corrosive resulting in the lead being leached from the pipes which causes a wide range of health concerns. Old homes can also contain asbestos, lead paint, high radon or carbon monoxide levels, and be poorly insulated and damp leading to mold and mildew. These problems can lead to cancer, asthma, kidney problems, neurological damage, and more. These old homes with these issues are more likely to be more affordable to someone on a lower income and they are generally located in neighborhoods with similar homes, leading to a vicious cycle of concentrated health issues. These neighborhoods are also disproportionately in areas with high levels of environmental hazards such as pollution, poor air quality, and other toxins. Similar to the cycle with education, we see a similar cycle in relation to housing: low income → affordable (and maybe poor quality) housing → health issues → compromised employment or unemployment.

Overcrowded conditions are known contributors to maintaining and complicating the eradication of various conditions such as skin infections, bacterial or viral infections, and eye disease. Overcrowded conditions can emerge due to people trying to save costs by living together but can also be cultural and a way to maintain family cohesion. There are social benefits to having family and others living together. Some people might think that less people living in a house is 'better', or that bigger houses are necessary. These value judgments are reflected in a range of policies such as child welfare that suggests maximum numbers of children in bedrooms and places restrictions on room sharing between children of various ages. A more culturally safe option would be to consult with families about preferred ways of living and to collaborate regarding housing design. Whether in urban or rural areas, knowing how people function in their homes is important to appropriate design.

Another area of concern in the U.S. is houselessness or homelessness. Some prefer the use of the term houselessness because though someone is not living in a house does not mean they do not have a home. Rather than learning just about how many people are homeless, ask yourself why are they homeless? What are the structural or personal contexts that lead to homelessness? There are enough houses empty in the U.S. for everyone to have a roof over their head.

As with education, the COVID-19 pandemic showed that policies and practices that were seen as acceptable now needed a major overhaul. For example, mortgage companies suddenly were able to be more lenient, landlords could not just evict people in the middle of a pandemic when people had lost their jobs and could not pay their rent. Suddenly, money was available for emergency relief. Not surprisingly, COVID-19 had a disproportionate impact on lower income people and their families while middle and higher income families with more secure housing even benefitted in the midst of a crisis. But the 'crisis' was arguably one that had always been there for low income, housing insecure, people and their families.

> **Reading**
> For a thorough read about the impact of toxic environments on human development and functioning, see Harriet Washington's meticulously researched book: Washington, H. A. (2019). *A terrible thing to Waste: Environmental racism and its assault on the American mind*. Little, Brown Spark.

> **Activity**
>
> What is the minimum wage for your state? Calculate how much income that equates to for a month. Search your local area for apartment or house rentals. You might use an app such as Trulia or Zillow. How much per month does a one or two-bedroom apartment cost? How much might you need to budget for transportation, whether that is public transportation, or a private car and car insurance and parking costs? What would you estimate food to cost per month? How about phone, internet, electricity, water, garbage, etc.? Could you afford to live independently on the minimum wage in your state or in your local area?

> **Films**
>
> *Cooked: Survival by Zip Code* is a PBS film about the 1995 heatwave in Chicago in which 739 people died of heat-related causes, most of them poor, elderly and African American.
>
> *Leave No Trace* is a 2018 film based on a true story about a veteran with PTSD living in the woods with his daughter in Oregon.

Racism and Discrimination

While there is substantial evidence to show that social and economic conditions contribute a great deal to health disparities between groups in the U.S., there is also a curious discrepancy—even when social and economic conditions are taken into consideration, the health and social conditions of particular groups in the U.S. are worse when compared to other groups.

To what do we attribute these differences? Historically, they were often attributed to biological differences, but we know that this explanation has no scientific basis. Could it be that poorer health and social outcomes are because, on the whole, healthcare providers provide poorer health care? Could it also be that the healthcare system disadvantages some groups (and privileges other groups) in systematic ways, or are there other factors at play?

Many terms exist enabling us to talk about or describe these differences in treatment and structures. While it is a good idea to understand this terminology, it is also important to remember that using some of these terms to describe people (for example, 'racist') can serve to perpetuate the very behaviors and attitudes that we are trying to stop.

Discrimination is when people treat other people differently (and unfavorably) because of their race, ethnicity, class, geographic location, mental status or substance issues, age, migration status, culture, religion, gender or sexual orientation. Racial discrimination is when people are treated differently because of presumed racial differences that are judged based on differences in skin color, hair, and other physical features.

Stereotyping, however, is when people use categories to create or maintain ideas about those categories. A *prejudice*, on the other hand, is making a judgment or holding a certain attitude (usually negative) about people based on their culture or identity. But if a person is prejudiced (holds attitudes or judgments) about certain groups, they do not necessarily discriminate (i.e., actions or behavior) against them.

Differences in healthcare treatment and structures that are due to or can be attributed to someone's ethnicity or race and that result in poorer outcomes can be described as *racist*. *Racism*, at an individual level, is when someone believes that people of a different 'race' are fundamentally inferior to those of another 'race'. '… Racism can be defined as phenomena that results in avoidable and unfair inequalities in power, resources and opportunities across racial or ethnic groups' (Berman & Paradies, 2010).

Privilege is about what others see in you. It's not about what you feel or understand about yourself. You may not come from a privileged background, but relative to another person, you may become privileged. For example, you may get served before someone because you are tall, or male or older or younger, or well-dressed. Privileges are the benefits someone gains from the ways in which they are perceived. Privilege is also ever-changing depending on the circumstances. Privilege is not a stable, enduring, or internal quality or characteristic.

Because of the complexities and diversity of people in racial and ethnic groups, and as a way to understand, for example, why there are health differences between groups of people, some researchers have looked to another concept—*visible minorities*. *Visible minorities* are people from non-dominant groups who are, in one way or another, 'visible' to the dominant population (Colic-Peisker, 2009). For example, Muslim women who veil would be visible minorities in a community where veiling is uncommon, but Muslim women who do not veil may not be 'visible' in the same sense in such communities. As for race or ethnicity, a Black American with dark skin would, according to this line of thinking, be more 'visible' (and therefore possibly a greater target for racial discrimination) than a Black American with lighter skin. It is an interesting concept that has not gone without criticism. The concept of visible minority is used widely in Canada and has come under attack from the United Nations as a concept that perpetuates racism (CBC News, 2007). The issue is complex, but certainly warrants discussion and debate.

Structural racism or *institutional racism* are the terms used to describe the systematic disadvantaging of racial and ethnic groups through systems or institutions or between institutions. This can include barriers (language, transport) or collective failure to provide appropriate services to people because of their race, culture, or ethnic origin. There is growing attention toward these concepts, and toward holding the systems or institutions responsible for their racist practices. For example, if a health service collects data that shows that overall, certain groups of patients received different treatment and that their health outcomes were worse compared to other patients, then the institution has a responsibility to modify its practices in order to achieve a more equitable outcome. Often, however, as with all forms of racism, structural or institutional racism can be difficult to identify.

As an example, consider that a lot of money and effort has gone toward smoking cessation campaigns and programs and smoking rates have decreased dramatically—but more so for certain groups of people—suggesting that the interventions have inadvertently disadvantaged particular groups and benefitted others, or that the information has not been effective for reducing smoking in certain groups. If the programs were designed by people from certain groups, then it should not be surprising that the interventions would benefit those groups and not others. This could be seen as an example of systemic racism, but the racism is in the processes and procedures and reflected through the outcomes.

Another important concept is that of internalized racism. *Internalized racism* is defined as 'the acceptance, by marginalized racial populations, of the negative societal beliefs and stereotypes about themselves' (Taylor & Grundy, 1996; Williams & Williams-Morris, 2000, p. 255). This acceptance can result in a 'self-fulfilling prophecy' of the beliefs and expectations of others. Internalized racism can also lead to rejection of culture and identity. While it is important to recognize internalized racism as an important part of the bigger picture of racism, we also need to be mindful of the possibility of *blaming the victim*.

This then brings us to the concept of *anti-racism*, which is more about what is done to actively combat racism. Anti-racism can include changing policies, providing anti-racism education or interventions, or 'anything that decreases the existence or practice of racism' (Paradies, 2007, p. 75).

> **Reading**
> Kendi, I. X. (2019). *How to be an anti-racist*. New York: One World, Random House.

In order to understand how, and if, racism or discrimination is at work in the U.S., we also need to understand the concepts of *equity* or *inequity* and *equality* or *inequality*. These are not the same things but are often used interchangeably. When we consider the gaps in life expectancy between various groups, this is an inequality—which relates to status, opportunity, or capacity (Leeder, 2003). However, *equity* has been defined as:

> … An ethical concept grounded in the principle of distributive justice … Equity in health reflects a concern to reduce unequal opportunities to be healthy [which are] associated with membership in less privileged social

groups, such as poor people; disenfranchised racial, ethnic or religious groups; women and rural residents.

... Pursuing equity in health means eliminating health disparities that are associated with underlying social disadvantage or marginalization. Equity ... focuses [our] attention on socially disadvantaged, marginalized or disenfranchised groups within and [among] countries, but not limited to the poor. (Braverman & Gruskin, 2003, as cited in Leeder, 2003)

Figure 7.2 illustrates the differences between equality, equity, reality, and liberation. As you can see, each person has the same size box regardless of the persons' height in the equality frame. We introduced this in chapter one. Everyone gets the same thing, it is equal, but not everyone can see the baseball game.

In the equity frame, we see that the shortest person gets two boxes, the middle person gets one box, and the tallest person doesn't get a box. Equity is based on fairness. They each get what they need to be able to see the baseball game. In the reality frame, we see that the tallest person has lots of boxes, even though they do not need them to be able to see the game. The middle-sized person has one box and can see the game, but the shortest person not only doesn't have a box but is in a hole!

How might that translate to reality as you know it? In the liberation frame, no one has a box because the fence has been removed! Did you even notice the fence? The fence in all of the other frames can signify sources of oppression. Liberation is about removing oppression. Kant (2015) proposes a liberation health framework that includes personal, cultural, and institutional factors that influence peoples' lives and identifying sources of oppression.

Activity

Can you think of another box or other experiences that could be depicted? Go to the website for Story Based Strategy, the 4th Box, for more activities and discussion around these boxes and think of possibilities for change. There is also a game app for your phone.

https://www.storybasedstrategy.org/the4thbox.

7 Determinants of Health   153

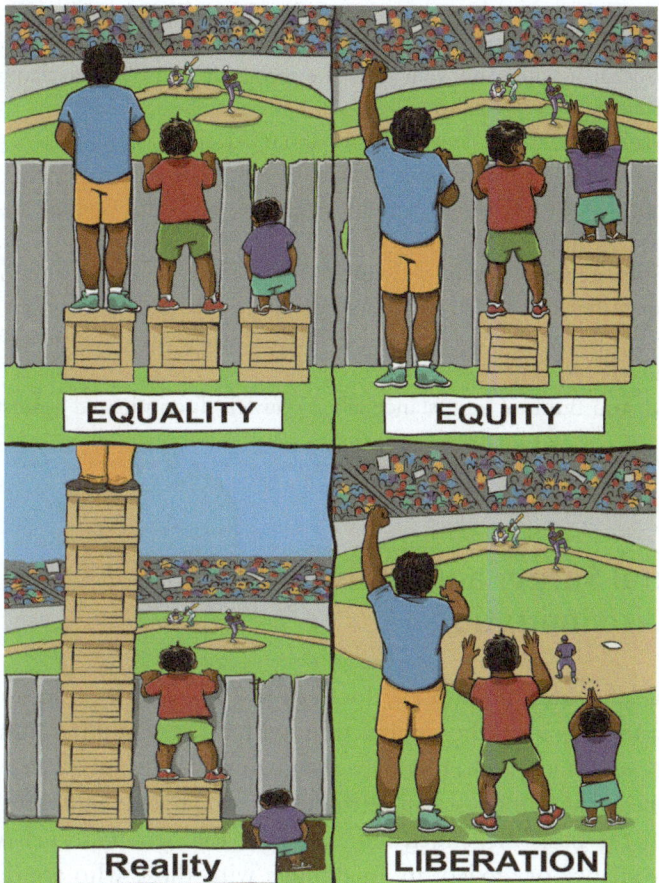

Fig. 7.2 A visual of the differences between equality, equity, reality and liberation (Image credit: #the4thbox Equality/Equity/Liberation image collaboration between *Center for Story-based Strategy* and *Interactive Institute for Social Change*. Reality panel created by Andrew Weizeman)

> **Scenario**
> A participant in a workshop shared her story of discrimination. As a Muslim woman, Amina chose to wear a headscarf when out in public. She described the open hostility and discriminatory treatment

> she received whenever she wore her scarf and eventually made a choice not to wear it when she went out. She recognized an obvious change in treatment for the better.
> - What messages did Amina receive about discrimination?
> - What did she have to do to reduce the risk of discrimination?
> - How do you feel about Amina's experience and what she has had to do to 'fit in'?
>
> In this scenario, Amina was able to make an external change in order to reduce her risk of being a target of discrimination. How might this make her feel and how might it be different when the discrimination is on the basis of skin color?
>
> Can you think of an instance when you felt discriminated against?

Cultural Safety and Racism and Discrimination

Cultural safety as a philosophy does not just ask health professionals to consider the impact of their interactions with those who differ from them on the basis of race. Cultural safety also requires professionals to examine their conscious or unconscious attitudes toward anyone who differs from them on the basis of gender, religion, age, abilities, or sexual orientation. Avoidance or anxiety in encounters with those who are different can be demonstrated through things like not looking at clients, cutting the consultation short, or providing less information than would be provided to others. These subtle differences can make a difference in health outcomes.

Health and human service professionals potentially hold great power over clients in their care. This power carries with it enormous responsibility. Understanding that power and reflecting on the historical and current abuses of this power relationship will hopefully help to improve care and reduce the current gaps in health that other measures have failed to reduce.

Some students find that learning about racism and discrimination brings out feelings of guilt or anger—guilt that maybe you or people close to you have intentionally or unintentionally treated people in discriminating ways, and anger that you are being, or might be, accused of behaving in such ways. However, learning about racism and discrimination for those in the psychology and health and human services field is critical. We know the impact of these elements on health and well-being. We all need to be able to examine the factors that influence our attitudes, assumptions, beliefs, behaviors and practices and, as professionals, taking responsibility for (and changing if necessary) these things that influence health and social care and their outcomes. Access to health and human services is more than just being able to get people through the door or having tokenistic artwork on the wall.

We all may be able to draw upon personal experiences of discrimination, and many of us may have actually been subjected to discriminatory policies that were sanctioned by law, as we saw in earlier chapters. For example, same-sex attracted people have been subjected to discriminatory laws and policies and, while some gains have been made toward equity, there are still areas in which the law discriminates.

It wasn't until 1964 with the Civil Rights Act and the passing of Medicare and Medicaid in 1965 that segregation in hospitals was prohibited. Health care for American Indian and Alaska Natives is provided through the Indian Health Service (IHS) but this is only provided on reservations and only a minority of AI/AN people live on or near reservations to gain access. Similarly, while many military veterans may access health care through the Veterans Administration (VA), not all are eligible for those services and complicated bureaucratic systems can significantly impact access.

Things taken for granted by many Americans, such as access to swimming pools, hotels, and cinemas have been legally denied to Indigenous Peoples and Black Americans until relatively recently. However, the changing of laws to prevent discrimination does not automatically remove discrimination; there are numerous examples today that are perhaps simply more covert in their implementation. For example, although segregation in a hospital would be unheard of today, have you, in your experiences in hospitals or medical clinics, ever noticed a separation, intentional or otherwise, of patients? The legal sanctions today, while possibly preventing overtly discriminating acts, may have inadvertently created a more subtle and covert kind of discrimination that is much harder to identify, label, and therefore prosecute.

Sexism and gender-based discrimination is another damaging aspect of daily interactions that have been difficult to fight. Read the following piece, identifying any elements of racism, sexism, and other forms of discrimination, while keeping in mind the impact of such experiences over a lifetime.

Scenario
Below is a true story by Chevara Orrin. Readers should be aware of the sensitive nature of the content of this story.

> I don't do it all the time. Only when I feel safe.
> And that shit's relative. Safety, I mean.

> First time, I was at a traffic light. It was early morning. Daybreak. They were gathered on the corner, at an intersection near my neighborhood. Day laborers waiting for a chance to work. A group of 20 or so. Smoking cigarettes. Shooting the breeze. I'd see them most days on my way to catch the sunrise over the St. Johns River.

> Usually, I don't get stopped by the light and turn before they even notice me.

> Not this morning.

> My ritual: convertible top down, meditation music on deck, water with fresh lemon, raw, unsalted almonds and a ripe banana.

> "Hey baby, I got something else to put in your mouth."

> I glance to my right. I say nothing but slowly lower the banana.

> "Yea YOU, sexy bitch!"

> The others laugh.

> I feel violated. Womanhood interrupted by the Patriarchy. I wonder how many seconds before the light turns green. I contemplate closing my convertible top.

I glance to my left. There's a gas station and sometimes police cars.

Not today.

A few moments later, the light changes and I drive away. I'm scared and pissed. I don't get far.

I've thought about it before. Exactly what I'd say. I even practiced in the mirror.

But each time, I'd freeze. Feeling overwhelmed with the ordinariness of it all.

Not today.

I abruptly turn around in the middle of the street, burning a little rubber.

There's an abandoned lot across the street from the day laborer spot and I pull in. I zig zag through oncoming traffic, my eyes focused on the one with the smart, dirty mouth.

They see me coming and give each other high fives.

I walk up, extend my hand.

"Hi, I'm Chevara. What's your name?"

He looks startled and grins. Like maybe I'm about to ask for his seven digits.

He says his name is T.J. I don't ask what it stands for. I don't care.

"I assume that what you were trying to do was say 'good morning' but somehow the right words failed you."

Before he has a chance to respond, I ask if he's ever heard of poet, essayist, and activist, June Jordan.

His blank stare answers my question before he begins to shake his head from left to right.

They've crowded around us now. It feels like spectator sport. I imagine I'm in a boxing ring. Except I'm not feeling much like a champ. I feel as though I might suffocate. I feel small. I'm wearing sneakers and not my trademark stilettos.

Spears of light pierce through clouds as the sky brightens and I feel a sliver of safety.

Before I lose my nerve, I tell him that June Jordan wrote a piece about Mike Tyson called "Requiem for a Champ." I read it in college.

She writes about the horrific conditions of poverty and oppression under which Tyson learned the "rules" of interacting with a girl...of talking...to a girl. I tell him that June Jordan says "the choices available to us dehumanize."

I'm not sure if he understands the quote or the enormity of the moment.

I ask him where he grew up, if he was raised with a momma, sisters, aunties or a grandmother. I ask if he has brothers, uncles, a dad or grandfather. I ask if he has daughters. He says his grandmother reared him. He says he grew up in the church and had a paper route. He says his little girl is three.

The other men are silent. A few have wandered away to stand on the periphery.

I tell him I live blocks away and that I shouldn't have to detour to feel safe. Not in my neighborhood nor anywhere in this world.

I tell him I'm an incest survivor. I ask them all if they know what that is. Now, it's really uncomfortable. A few lower their heads. One nods.

"It means that my father's semen was on my thigh when I was 10."

I say it slowly. I want them to hear it. I want them to feel the pain in my words.

I tell him that his morning greeting almost f***** up my day. Disrupted my spirit. That his words felt violent and hurtful and disrespectful and mostly made me sad.

Something changes. The air is lighter and heavier at the same time. He looks like he might cry.

He tells me again that his daughter is three. He calls her name.

I tell him that I don't need him to see me as his mother or sister or daughter. I need him to see me as human.

He asks if he can give me a hug. I walk into his outstretched arms.

I leave him with June Jordan, whispering: "I can stop whatever violence starts with me."

I don't do it all the time. Only when I feel safe.

And that shit's relative. Safety, I mean.

I've done it with construction workers at a city job site and college students in a grocery store near the frozen waffles and corporate executives in a towering office complex.

Irrespective of status or profession or age or geography.

The struggle is real. The intersection of my identity as a Black woman.

The struggle is real. Navigating toxic masculinity on a daily.

The struggle is real. Layers of unbalanced power and complicity of men in causing harm and maintaining misogynistic structures.

The struggle is real. Demanding autonomy of voice and power of agency in a world filled with men who never learned how to talk to a girl.

Today, I awakened channeling June Jordan's spirit:

"...I am the history of battery assault and limitless armies against whatever I want to do with my mind and my body and my soul...

...and I can't tell you who the hell set things up like this but I can tell you that from now on my resistance my simple and daily and nightly self-determination may very well cost you your life."

I don't do it all the time. Only when I feel safe.

And that shit's relative. Safety, I mean.

I am not the one. I believe in necessary disruptions. You will be held accountable on my watch (Fig. 7.3).

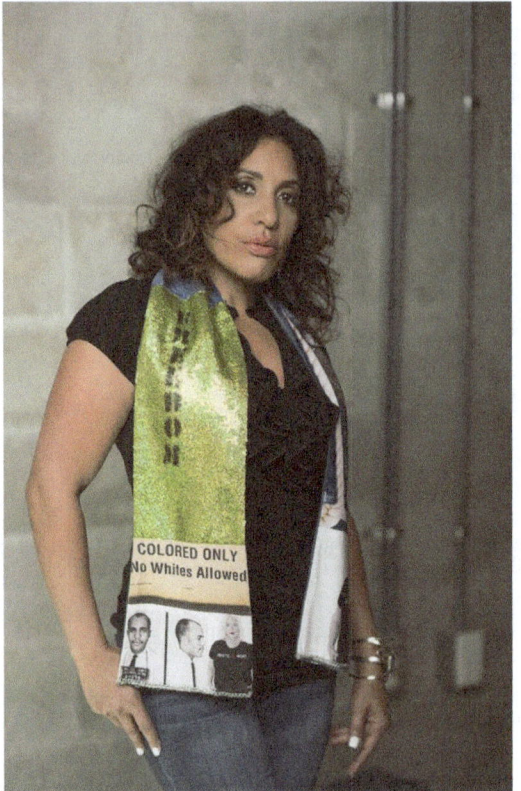

Fig. 7.3 Chevara Orrin

**I received a few questions and comments about the scarf I'm wearing. I'll provide context.

The scarf is from the Freedom Collection that I created in collaboration with fiber artist, Laurie Phoenix Niewidok, that honors the Freedom Riders of the 1960s.

Art is often an access point. Connecting us despite of, and because of, our differences. Engaging even the most cynical among us. Throughout the ages, artists have used canvas to create social and political change. Artists have used prose to record memories, resist oppression and inspire revolutions. Artists have danced for freedom and awakened us to the realities of racial injustice. There is redemptive power in the voice of the artist.

My father (whose image is on the scarf next to my white, Jewish mother) was on the first bus that arrived in Jackson, MS on May 24, 1961. The "colored only" sign is reminiscent of Jim Crow laws that mandated the segregation of public schools, public places, and public transportation, and the segregation of restrooms, restaurants, and drinking fountains for whites and blacks. Facilities for Black people were consistently inferior and underfunded, compared to the facilities for white Americans; sometimes there were no Black facilities.

My father, James Bevel initiated, strategized, directed, and developed SCLC's three major successes of the Civil Rights era: the 1963 Birmingham Children's Crusade, the 1965 Selma voting rights movement, and the 1966 Chicago open housing movement. Grammy and Academy award-winning artist, Common portrays my father in the critically acclaimed film, *Selma*.

My father is also perpetrator of my incest.

Jim Crow:

https://m.youtube.com/watch?v=wL2gjxx9qa4.

My father:

https://breachofpeace.com/blog/?p=85.

Incest trial: Carpenter, L. (2008, May 25). A Father's Shadow: He was a hero of the civil rights movement, but he was something else too—A man who preyed on his daughters. *Washington Post*, p. W16, accessed 4 November 2020 from

https://www.washingtonpost.com/wp-dyn/content/story/2008/05/22/ST2008052 202216.html?noredirect=on&fbclid=IwAR2Hv4TX28XCwYREsext9vwtp6-2cy 4nE7y4lAXyd58n5Bt0iQZWmm4WI0c.

> **Critical Thinking**
> - What can we learn from Chevara's story about intergenerational trauma? The impacts of harm continue, whether those traumas relate to any part of our identities, we see in this story how 'hurt people, hurt people'.
> - Previously, we discussed diunital logic. How can this be applied to Chevara's relationship with her father? She can appreciate that her father was an important part of the civil rights movement and also that he hurt her and his other daughters.
> - 'I don't need him to see me as his mother or sister or daughter. I need him to see me as human'. What does this line say to you about cultural safety?

> **Making It Local**
> What examples, if any, can you identify from your internships, placements, or experiences at health services of possible systemic bias or institutional racism?
>
> What, if any, racial tensions or issues are current in the areas where you live or work? You might find these in your local newspaper.

Conclusion

We have explored how to examine the impact of dominant cultures on non-dominant cultures and how we might diminish any potential harm that results. Cultural safety requires professionals to examine any taken-for-granted place of privilege and the realities of racism and discrimination in order to challenge these in professional practice. Health and human services professionals can only hope to play a role in closing the gaps in the health and social outcomes by considering *all* determinants of health: biological, psychological, social, political, spiritual, and cultural.

References

Angelou, M. (1986). *All god's children need traveling shoes*. Random House.
Berman, G., & Paradies, Y. (2010). Racism, disadvantage and multiculturalism: Towards effective anti-racist praxis. *Ethnic and Racial Studies, 33*, 214–232.
CBC News. (2007, 8 March). *Term 'visible minorities' may be discriminatory, UN body warns Canada*. CBC News. https://www.cbc.ca/news/canada/term-visible-minorities-may-be-discriminatory-un-body-warns-canada-1.690247.
CDC. (n.d.). *About the social determinants of health*. https://www.cdc.gov/socialdeterminants/about.html.
Colic-Peisker, V. (2009). Visibility, settlement success and life satisfaction in three refugee communities in Australia. *Ethnicities, 9*(2), 175–199.
Dawes, D. E. (2020). *The political determinants of health*. Johns Hopkins University Press.
Kant, J. D. (2015). Towards a socially just social work practice: The liberation health model. *Critical and Radical Social Work, 3*, 309–319.
Knibb-Lamouche, J. (2012). Culture as a social determinant of health. In *Roundtable on the Promotion of Health Equity and the Elimination of Health Disparities; Board on Population Health and Public Health Practice*. Institute of Medicine. National Academies Press (US); 2013 December 19. https://www.ncbi.nlm.nih.gov/books/NBK201298/.
Leeder, S. (2003). Achieving equity in the Australian healthcare system. *Medical Journal of Australia, 179*, 475–478.
Marmot, M. (2015). *The health gap: The challenge of an unequal world*. Bloomsbury.
Paradies, Y. (2007). Racism. In B. Carson, T. Dunbar, R. Chenhall, & R. Bailie (Eds.), *Social determinants of indigenous health* (pp. 65–86). Sydney: Allen and Unwin.
Reid, J. B., & Taylor, K. (2011). Indigenous mind: A framework for culturally safe Indigenous health research and practice. *Aboriginal and Islander*

Health Worker Journal, 35(4), 4–6. https://search.informit.org/doi/10.3316/informit.357506114954970.

Taylor, J., & Grundy, C. (1996). Measuring Black internalization of White stereotypes about African Americans: The Nadanolitization Scale. In R. L. Jones (Ed.), *Handbook of tests and measurements of Black populations* (Vol. 2, pp. 217–226). Cobb & Henry.

Taylor, K., & Thompson-Guerin, P. (2019). *Health Care and Indigenous Australians: Cultural safety in practice* (3rd ed.). Red Globe Press. ISBN-13: 9781352005424.

WHO. (2008). *The commission on the social determinants of health—What, why and how*. https://www.who.int/social_determinants/thecommission/finalreport/about_csdh/en/.

WHO. (2011). *Rio political declaration on social determinants of health*. https://www.who.int/sdhconference/declaration/en/.

WHO. (n.d.). *Social determinants of health*. https://www.who.int/health-topics/social-determinants-of-health#tab=tab_1.

Williams, D. R., & Williams-Morris, R. (2000). Racism and mental health: The African American experience. *Ethnicity & Health, 5,* 243–268. https://doi.org/10.1080/713667453.

8

Stats and Maps

In this chapter, *Stats and Maps*, we explore various sources of information that can be helpful to our learning and understanding about culture and diversity. We will examine the roles of epidemiology and human geography and discuss some of the limitations and pitfalls of large-scale data. We explore some of the myths and stereotyped ideas that can interfere with culturally safe practice and attempt to counter some of the misconceptions with an overview of the demographic and health statistics. We also consider the use of maps as sources of information.

Chapter Objectives

After completing this chapter, you should be able to:

- identify sources of demographic and health information
- understand the use of maps as sources of information for understanding health and well-being

- understand the value and limitations of statistical information in health and human service delivery.

Awareness

We learned earlier in this book about the cyclical nature of the components required for culturally safe practice. One component of culturally safe practice is cultural awareness, including self-awareness. Awareness of differences and also commonalities is essential for culturally safe practice. We already learned about the importance of historical differences between groups of people and how those histories influence contemporary health and well-being and the delivery of health care and other human services. We'll now look at information, such as statistics and maps, that we might access to inform our understanding of disparities in health and well-being. We've also briefly discussed how data only provide us with part of the story.

Culturally safe practice requires ongoing learning. Remember, culturally safe practice does not end at awareness, but is just one part of the process. The more we learn about ourselves and who we are, we gain an appreciation for the complexity and diversity of those in our care. In that spirit, let's explore some sources of information that can help us to understand ourselves and others and how to use that information in culturally safe ways.

Epidemiology and COVID-19

Epidemiology is the field of health and medicine that studies and analyzes health-related conditions and diseases in populations. Epidemiologists study the incidence and prevalence of illnesses and other health-related events. Incidence is the number or rate of new cases while prevalence is the number or rate of an illness or condition in a population at a particular point in time or period of time. For example, during the COVID-19 pandemic, the number of daily new cases reflected the incidence, while prevalence would reflect the total number of people currently sick with COVID-19.

> **Website**
> For a brief history of the beginnings of modern epidemiology, read the story of John Snow provided at the link below. This overview describes how Western medicine has theorized health in the past and that what is commonly accepted today was thought too radical to be believed.
> Vachon, D. (n.d.). *Doctor John Snow blames water pollution for cholera epidemic*. UCLA Department of Epidemiology. https://www.ph.ucla.edu/epi/snow/fatherofepidemiology.html.

We can further understand health and illness by looking at the distribution of an illness such as the frequency or locations or other patterns that indicate where an illness is more likely to occur or population groups more at risk. Using COVID-19 as an example again, collecting and analyzing the age, gender, and race of those who got sick was critically important to understand how the virus was spreading and who was more likely to be affected (risk). The elderly and those with pre-existing health conditions were found to be most at risk. Additionally, following cases geographically, informed quarantine and lockdown decisions as a way to help reduce the spread.

While the number of cases and deaths from COVID-19 was attracting a great deal of attention, it became apparent that collecting and reporting on hospitalization numbers was also critical. Most people could test positive for COVID-19 (a case), yet never get sick enough to go to the hospital. While knowing the number of cases lets us know how the virus was spreading, it didn't tell us the whole story. It was also important to know how many people were getting so sick that they required hospitalization so that hospitals could plan and be prepared. The COVID-19 pandemic exposed some of the harshest realities of who we are as a nation and became politically and socially divisive.

The dominance of the biomedical model in our country quickly became more apparent as strategies were swiftly employed to isolate and quarantine and billions were spent on testing, developing, and delivering a vaccine. The problems with our healthcare system, and the disaster of linking health insurance through employment were quickly apparent as businesses closed down and people lost their jobs and health insurance. As already discussed, the pandemic also exposed weaknesses in housing and education.

With COVID-19 impacting people with pre-existing health conditions, our continued failure to create healthy environments and prevent chronic health conditions was undeniable. At the time of writing, it is still unclear the full damage the epidemic had on our nation, our communities, families, and individuals. We will hopefully learn from the experiences and enact sustainable changes that create a more equitable, healthy society for all.

Life Expectancy

Generally, health status and outcomes for health are measured and determined through a wide range of sources and types of information. For example, life expectancy is a statistic that indicates the number of years a person can expect to live, on average. Disparities, or differences, in life expectancy between various groups can indicate disparities in access to health care, the quality of living and working environments, and indicate inequalities in incomes. Clearly there are a number of factors relevant to understanding this measure, but the important thing to know as professionals (unless you are specializing in life expectancy) is that there are huge disparities in life expectancy between groups.

> **Reading**
> See this article for some in-depth exploration of racial and ethnic differences in life expectancy in the U.S.
> Cantu, P. A., Hayward, M. D., Hummer, R. A., & Chiu, C. T. (2013). New estimates of racial/ethnic differences in life expectancy with chronic morbidity and functional loss: Evidence from the National

Health Interview Survey. *Journal of Cross-cultural Gerontology, 28*(3), 283–297. https://doi.org/10.1007/s10823-013-9206-5.

Life expectancy is a statistical measure that is often used to assess or compare the health of populations. This can be measured in a few different ways. Life expectancy at birth is probably the most common measure and can be measured by cohort or period. For example, cohort life expectancy takes into consideration that someone born in the 1940s may not have the same life expectancy as someone born in the 1990s. Period life expectancy is the measure commonly used by agencies and organizations. Life expectancy numbers can be used to guide policy and funding decisions as well as planning for care needs.

> **Activity**
> Look at this interactive map for life expectancy in the U.S. from the National Center for Health Statistics: https://www.cdc.gov/nchs/data-visualization/life-expectancy/. This map allows the user to drill down to census tract level. Users can also explore data by state and county and enter specific addresses. For example, users can see that in some Census tracts in Delaware County, Pennsylvania, the life expectancy is as low as 67 years, but only a few short miles away, the life expectancy is as high as 86 years, with a state average of 78.6 years. At the state level, we can see that Mississippi has a life expectancy of 74.9, while life expectancy in California is 81.3 years. Within Mississippi, life expectancy is just 59.5 years in Harrison County, and is 26 years higher in Coahoma County at 85.5 years. Explore the map for the statistics on life expectancy in your area. What have you learned about how your area compares to neighboring communities or the state?
>
> But how do we interpret this information? What does it mean when life expectancy is so extremely different among people who live just a few miles from each other?

We can look at life expectancy between groups of people, such as that shown in Fig. 8.1. This figure shows that, overall (on average), women live longer than men, in any group. We also see a large disparity in life expectancy between groups (on average), with Black Americans living shorter lives and Hispanic American living longer. These large-scale data can be useful in drawing our attention to *something*, but we also need to be mindful that these numbers do not represent a *person*.

Other data and measures for understanding health status and health outcomes are to look at morbidity and mortality (death) rates; self-assessed health; disabilities; low birth weight; maternal mortality rate and other birth and pregnancy outcomes; and various health service information (such as hospitalizations). It is important to recognize that sometimes we have the data to show there are differences between groups, but these data do not necessarily tell us *why* there are differences. It is in the interpretation of the data that we have to be very careful.

So, what do these statistics mean? Why do some groups die earlier than others from the same condition? Are they receiving different, and maybe worse, health care? Why are some babies more likely to die? While it

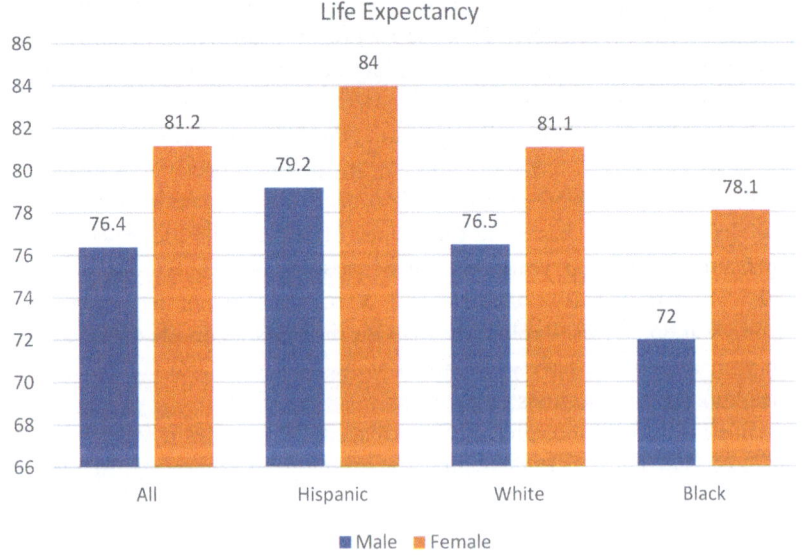

Fig. 8.1 Life expectancy for male and female and White, Black, and Hispanic (*Source* Arias, 2016)

might be desirable to have simple answers to these questions, the reality is that there are no simple answers. Be wary of reports or publications that attempt to simplify the answers down to abstract or generalized conclusions. For example, we might say that higher suicide rates are the result of loss of identity related to loss of land, culture, and traditions. But what does that really mean in practice and how can you, as a professional, do something about it? Similarly, we might say that there are 'barriers to accessing health care', which is why some groups are more likely to die from conditions at a younger age. But what exactly are these barriers and how do we alleviate them?

All of this suggests that while statistics have a valuable role to play in identifying issues of concern, they need to be interrogated to ensure they do not distort the realities on the ground. Also, statistics, even those shared here, need to be used cautiously. Imagine attending a lecture or conference where you and your family were portrayed as likely to die younger, likely to develop a range of chronic diseases, likely to be incarcerated or whatever the interpretation of the data suggested. What impact might that have on your own well-being? Health statistics represent groups of people, and no singular person in particular. When using such information in practice, it is important to be sensitive. A colleague watching a presentation on life expectancies noted his own ethnic group on the graph, and said, 'I should be dead by now. Maybe I should retire'. How might information be shared with individuals and groups in a culturally safe way?

Demographic Profile

While epidemiology specifically focuses on health issues and illnesses, demography is the statistical study of populations in general such as births, deaths, marriages, or various descriptions of the population as a whole; the kind of information collected, analyzed, and reported with the census. Populations can be viewed by age, race or ethnicity, gender, religion, etc.

Human geography is the study of relationships between people and places, such as migration patterns. Having an understanding of human geography helps us to understand who we are and how we fit in to our local and wider communities, as well as understanding who are the populations we are serving as health and human services professionals.

> **Activity**
> Think about some of the characteristics of your own identity. How does who you are fit into the patterns of populations in your area? Before going to the statistics, take a moment to write down your current beliefs about the identities of people who live in your town, county, or state. A good first place to look is the U.S. Census Quick Stats for data on your local area. What have you learned about yourself or the people who make up your communities? Explore various topics for your immediate or larger area. You might want to explore variables such as age, gender, religion, disability, ethnic or racial identity, sexual orientation, and socioeconomic variables such as home ownership, education levels, poverty levels, and employment.
> - How do the demographics of your location differ from your state or the overall U.S. population?
> - Look at various statistics such as the actual number versus the proportion of the population. What relevance might these numbers have?

Let's look at an example for the American Indian and Alaska Native population. Table 8.1 shows that 1.7% of the U.S. population identified as American Indian or Alaska Native (AI/AN) in the 2010 Census (Census, 2012) and includes 5.2 million people. If you were to allocate funding based on numbers alone, how would this information inform your decisions? Numbers are not always a good indicator of need. What information do we need to make different decisions about allocation of funding or healthcare and human services needs?

Where do you think the majority of the AI/AN population live in the U.S.? Which states do you think have the highest AI/AN population? The numbers alone are not the whole story but are part of the story and may lead to asking more questions. Such as, where are the greatest number of hospitalizations among AI/AN populations? Is this enough

Table 8.1 American Indian and Alaska Native population (alone or in combination) by state and (% of total 2010 state population)

State	AI/AN	State	AI/AN	State	AI/AN
Alabama	57,118 (1.2)	Louisiana	55,079 (1.2)	Oklahoma	482,760 (12.9)
Alaska	138,312 (19.5)	Maine	18,482 (1.4)	Oregon	109,223 (2.9)
Arizona	353,386 (5.5)	Maryland	58,657 (1.0)	Pennsylvania	81,092 (0.6)
Arkansas	47,588 (1.6)	Massachusetts	50,705 (0.8)	Rhode Island	14,394 (1.4)
California	723,225 (1.9)	Michigan	139,095 (1.4)	South Carolina	42,171 (0.9)
Colorado	107,832 (2.1)	Minnesota	101,900 (1.9)	South Dakota	82,073 (10.0)
Connecticut	31,140 (0.9)	Mississippi	25,910 (0.9)	Tennessee	54,874 (0.9)
Delaware	9,899 (1.1)	Missouri	72,376 (1.2)	Texas	315,264 (1.3)
District of Columbia	6,521 (1.0)	Montana	78,601 (7.9)	Utah	50,064 (1.8)
Florida	162,562 (0.9)	Nebraska	29,816 (1.6)	Vermont	7,379 (1.2)
Georgia	84,024 (0.9)	Nevada	55,945 (2.0)	Virginia	80,924 (1.0)
Hawaii	33,470 (2.5)	New Hampshire	10,524 (0.8)	Washington	198,998 (3.0)
Idaho	36,385 (2.3)	New Jersey	70,716 (0.8)	West Virginia	13,314 (0.7)
Illinois	101,451 (0.8)	New Mexico	219,512 (10.7)	Wisconsin	86,228 (1.5)
Indiana	49,738 (0.8)	New York	221,058 (1.1)	Wyoming	18,596 (3.3)
Iowa	24,511 (0.8)	North Carolina	184,082 (1.9)	Puerto Rico	35,753 (1.0)
Kansas	59,130 (2.0)	North Dakota	42,996 (6.4)	Total U.S. alone or in combination	5.2 million (1.7)
Kentucky	31,355 (0.7)	Ohio	90,124 (0.8)	Total U.S. alone	2.9 million (0.9)

Source U.S. Census Bureau (2011, 2012)

now to decide where funding should be allocated? What about those who don't get to access health services, or who don't even get counted in the data collection?

Statistics can answer specific questions such as how many, what proportion, and so on, but more information is needed to interpret and analyze the data. For example, in the report 'Twice Invisible, Understanding rural Native America' (Dewees & Marks, 2017) researchers note that outdated definitions and poor data quality have led to misunderstandings about Native Americans and rural America. Specifically, with their re-analysis of data, they found that the oft-cited information that the majority of Native Americans live in urban areas is wrong and that, in fact, most Native Americans live in rural or small-town areas or in or near reservations.

> **Activity**
> - Study the information presented in Table 8.1. What states have the largest numbers of AI/AN by number? What states have the highest proportion of AI/AN? Look at the information for your own state. Were these numbers surprising to you?
> - Is there a Federally Recognized Tribe or State Recognized Tribe in your state? Why might this be important? See the National Congress of American Indians website for information and resources about Tribal Recognition in the U.S. https://www.ncai.org/about-tribes.

Urban, Suburban, Rural

As we continue to build our awareness, of self and of others, let's now look at where people live and why and when that might matter as health and human services professionals. Where do people live in the U.S. and how does this impact culture, identity, health behaviors, and healthcare access and outcomes? What could be important for us to understand as health and human services professionals when it comes to these varying contexts?

People living in rural areas in the U.S. generally experience greater health disparities when compared to people living in urban or suburban areas. In general, life expectancy is lower, mortality rates are higher, and diseases and disabilities are higher in rural areas. People in rural areas are more geographically isolated which can mean accessing health care and other services can be much more difficult. Employment and educational opportunities can also be more limited.

> **Resources**
> See the Rural Health Information Hub for information about rural health in the U.S. including statistics, how to find statistics, data visualizations and maps: https://www.ruralhealthinfo.org/.
> See this Pew Research Center report, May 2018, *What unites and divides urban, suburban and rural communities*: https://www.pewsocialtrends.org/2018/05/22/what-unites-and-divides-urban-suburban-and-rural-communities/.

Table 8.2 shows the geographic distribution of healthcare professionals. Importantly, this table shows that the distribution of the health workforce is not aligned with the distribution of the U.S. population. For example, while 20% of the U.S. population live in rural or remote areas, only 11% of physicians are in those areas. While more primary care professionals are in rural areas compared to specialists, they are still more concentrated in urban areas.

> **Resources**
> American Medical Association, *Health Workforce Mapper*: The AMA Health Workforce Mapper is a free, customizable, interactive tool that illustrates the geographic distribution of the health care workforce. https://www.ama-assn.org/about/research/health-workforce-mapper.

Table 8.2 Geographic distribution of healthcare professionals, 2010 (%)

Geography	All specialties			Primary care					U.S. population
	NP	PA	Physicians	NP	PA	Family physicians/GPs	General Internal medicine	General pediatrics	
Urban	84.4	84.4	89.0	72.2	75.1	77.5	89.8	91.2	80
Large rural	8.9	8.8	7.1	11.0	11.7	11.1	6.7	6.2	10
Small rural	3.9	3.8	2.6	7.7	6.9	7.2	2.4	1.8	5
Remote rural/frontier	2.8	3.0	1.3	9.1	6.3	4.2	1.1	0.8	5

Source Agency for Healthcare Research and Quality (2018)

> **Film and Website**
> Watch the documentary *Remote Area Medical* and view their website for information about their work and how to sign up to volunteer: https://www.ramusa.org/.
> - What other barriers can you identify that would prevent certain populations from accessing health care?
> - What strategies could overcome some of the barriers identified?

Age Distributions

One way we can understand the health and well-being and other social issues for a community is to explore the age distribution within that community. Age is not distributed in the same ways for different groups. Perhaps large families may be more likely in some communities compared to others.

Table 8.3 shows the median age of males and females in various population groups from the 2019 Census Annual Estimates (U.S. Census, 2020). These data show us that the median age for White Americans (39.5) is higher compared to all the other groups and is nearly 10 years higher than for Native Hawaiian/Pacific Islander Americans. Median age can be a useful simple indicator of how youthful a particular population is or how much that population is aging. But we might want to know

Table 8.3 Median age by sex and race in the U.S

	Male	Female	Total
Black	30.6	34.1	32.3
AI/AN	30.5	32.1	31.3
Asian	33.7	36.3	35.0
NHPI	29.1	30.1	29.6
White	38.3	40.8	39.5

Source https://www.census.gov/data/tables/time-series/demo/popest/2010s-national-detail.html (Median age and age by sex, race, and Hispanic origin, 2019. This table shows total race which includes Hispanic for each of the race groups)

more detail about how a population is distributed. For this, we might use population pyramids.

Figure 8.2 depicts the population pyramids showing that there are very different age structures between these selected population groups which include Native Hawaiian/ Pacific Island (NHPI), Asian, American Indian/Alaska Native (AI/AN), Black and White. Schaeffer (2019) shows that the most common age among Whites is 58, which is more than double that for racial and ethnic minorities.

Activity Why Do Population Structures Matter?
- Do you notice anything startling from the population pyramids? Look at the proportion of ages in these populations. Which groups have the most people older than 55 years? Which groups have the least? Which groups have a greater proportion under 24? What impact might these differences have on these populations?

Think about the current age criteria for retirement in the U.S. Generally, this is about 65 years old. If life expectancy for many groups in the U.S. is known to be significantly less than average, how might the criteria for retirement actually disadvantage certain groups, such as those living in poverty? Is there any argument for an adjustment or is equal treatment actually equitable? Are there other age-related policies that you can think of that might lead to inequities given these population variations? How might health and social outcomes be related to these population structures and variations?

Critical Thinking
- Who are the dominant institutions that collect and disseminate population health data?
- What worldview or philosophical perspectives inform the data collection, interpretation, and dissemination?
- How do the data and information we have access to paint a deficit picture of certain groups?

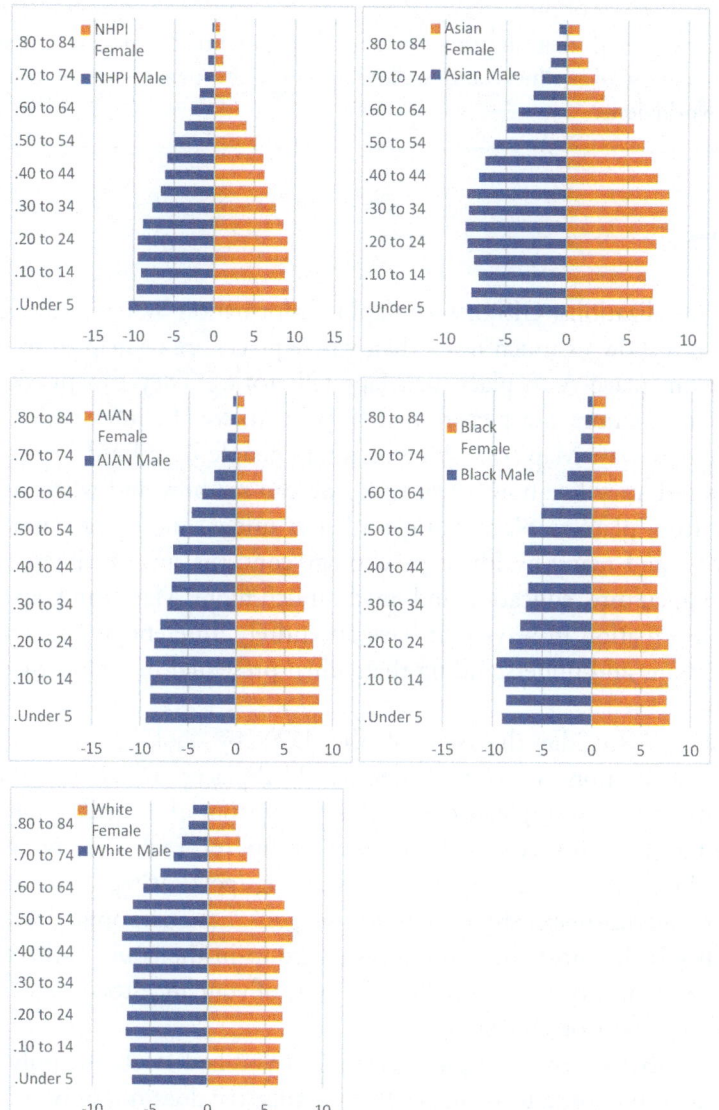

Fig. 8.2 Population pyramids for Native Hawaiian and Pacific Islanders (NHPI), Asian, AI/AN, Black and White males and females in the U.S.

> - How could that information and data potentially conceal understanding of wellness and well-being from the perspective of other worldviews?

Maps

Data visualizations, GIS or Geographic Information Systems, and other maps can show us much more than where places are or help us to navigate from place A to place B. Maps tell stories. They can provide us with information in a picture that helps us to see the information in a whole new way. Maps can show us where people have lived in the past and where they live now. Over time, we can see how and when people move from place to place and get a better understanding of migration, identity, and many health or psychology concerns such as illness, jobs, housing, culture, education and much, much more. Maps can help us to 'see' information in ways that have an entirely different impact on our perceptions and understanding than when presented in a table or other graphs.

We can see the diversity of the U.S. by looking at maps or data visualizations of Native identity, birthplaces, racial, or cultural identities. For example, explore this map from the *Washington Post* showing the most common ancestry group for each county in the U.S. https://www.washingtonpost.com/blogs/govbeat/wp/2014/04/18/ethnic-america-mapped-your-countys-biggest-ancestral-populations/.

What is the most common ancestry group in the county where you live? Did that surprise you? Where do some of your ancestors come from? Do they appear on this map?

Most people have multiple ancestries. If you had to choose only one, how do you choose to identify? If your ancestry does not appear, what might that indicate? As with most information, when we start to look more closely, we might find that we have even more questions and questions that we didn't even realize were questions.

Statisticians are constantly having to make decisions about what information to include or exclude and how to categorize or summarize data so that it makes sense. We also might wonder about the quality of the data. We are assuming that everyone who answers ancestry questions are answering 'honestly' or 'truthfully', but have you ever had the experience of changing how you might answer questions about identity? Maybe in some contexts you provide certain answers, but in other contexts, you provide a different answer. That doesn't mean that you were dishonest. To create an ancestry map such as the one above, people had to answer questions about ancestry. Many things can influence how a person answers those questions as discussed in the chapter about history. There have been many groups throughout history that have been discriminated against and would therefore have good reasons to change the ancestry they identify with, if at all possible. Keep in mind as a health or human services professional that some clients may well hesitate to answer such questions due to these histories and even current political or other issues.

Websites

Here are a number of websites with various forms of data visualization and maps that tell a story about significant events that have shaped our country and therefore the health or ill-health of our people, particularly Black and Indigenous people. For example, in the History chapter we talked about the history of segregation, but have you thought about how segregation might look today? What other maps or data visualizations can you find for health or population issues of interest to you?

Here are some maps showing segregation and integration and diversity:

- University of Iowa, *Placing Segregation* project, Explores spatial patterns of residential segregation in Washington, DC, Omaha Nebraska, and Nashville Tennessee: https://dsps.lib.uiowa.edu/placingsegregation/.
- University of Virginia, Racial Dot map of the 2010 census: https://demographics.coopercenter.org/racial-dot-map.
- National Geographic race, ethnicity, diversity in the U.S. interactive map: https://www.nationalgeographic.com/magazine/2018/10/diversity-race-ethnicity-united-states-america-interactive-map/.

- *Washington Post*: Segregation in U.S. Cities interactive map: https://www.washingtonpost.com/graphics/2018/national/segregation-us-cities/.

The following are a few maps and resources relating to historical events such as slavery, emancipation, and lynching.

- These maps from the *Smithsonian Magazine* show how slavery expanded across the United States. https://www.smithsonianmag.com/history/maps-reveal-slavery-expanded-across-united-states-180951452/.
- *Civil War Washington* examines the U.S. national capital from multiple perspectives as a case study of social, political, cultural, and medical/scientific transitions provoked or accelerated by the Civil War. The project draws on the methods of many fields to create a digital resource that chronicles the war's impact on the city. https://civilwardc.org/.
- The University of Richmond in Virginia created the *Visualizing Emancipation* website that explores the more complicated process of emancipation through a series of events and interactions between federal policies, armies in the field and actions of enslaved men and women. https://dsl.richmond.edu/emancipation/.
- *Lynching in America* is a project by the Equal Justice Initiative https://lynchinginamerica.eji.org/. This website includes stories, videos and interactive maps about the 4,000 lynchings in the U.S. between 1877 and 1950 and the Great Migration.
- *Mapping the Stacks*, http://mts.lib.uchicago.edu/ is a University of Chicago project that aims to identify and organize uncatalogued archival collections that chronicle Black Chicago between the 1930s and 1970s, in order to increase their use by researchers and the general public. The project includes various kinds of artifacts: literary manuscripts and visual illustrations; rare books and home movies; correspondence and photographs; ephemera and tape-recorded sound.
- The University of Delaware, *The Colored Conventions Project* is a collaborative project that brings nineteenth-century Black organizing to digital life through convention records and exhibits. https://coloredconventions.org/.

Below is a list of maps relating to Native American diversity and languages.

- Wang, H. L. (2014). *The map of Native American tribes you've never seen before*. NPR. https://www.npr.org/sections/codeswitch/2014/06/24/323665644/the-map-of-native-american-tribes-youve-never-seen-before.
- Sturtevant, W. C., & U. S. Geological Survey. (1967). *National atlas. Indian tribes, cultures & languages: United States*. Reston, VA: Interior, Geological Survey. [Map] Library of Congress. https://www.loc.gov/item/95682185/.
- *Native Lands*, crowd-sourced global interactive map: https://native-land.ca/. Check out your location on this map to find out the Indigenous groups for the land that you live on.
- 1881 Map of Linguistic Stocks of American Indians Library of Congress https://www.loc.gov/item/2001620496/. This map is an interesting look at the diversity of Indigenous languages.

Below are a few maps relating to religions in the U.S.

- The Religious States of American in 22 Maps, *The Washington Post*. https://www.washingtonpost.com/blogs/govbeat/wp/2015/02/26/the-religious-states-of-america-in-22-maps/.
- The Pew Research Center has an interactive map for religions in the U.S. https://www.pewforum.org/religious-landscape-study/.

This *Smithsonian Magazine* map shows queer geography over time in the U.S.

- *Smithsonian Magazine*, this interactive map visualizes the Queer geography of the 20th Century; *Mapping the Gay Guides* visualizes local queer spaces' evolution between 1965 and 1980. https://www.smithsonianmag.com/history/interactive-map-visualizes-queer-geography-20th-century-america-180974306/.

Critical Thinking About the Statistics: Identity

The categories of 'race' and ethnicity have gone through many changes. For example, the 'one drop rule' or the 'one Black ancestor rule' implied that if a person had even 'one drop' of Black ancestry they would be identified as Black. This 'rule' was able to be exploited by plantation owners or others looking to maintain high numbers of those they enslaved. Different states at various times altered or modified the requirements for Black identification also showing how random and unscientific the notion was. But ask yourself this: if your identity, as indicated by checking a box on a form, could result in enslavement on the one hand, or freedom on the other, which box would you check, if you could?

On the other hand, Native American identity has been (and continues to be) subjected to the opposite rule. That is, minimum 'blood quantums' are required to be legally considered Native American and to gain membership in various tribes (and therefore, access to various resources). Why might minimum blood quantums be required for Native American identity (with increasing requirements over time), but the opposite true for Black Americans (albeit, in the past)?

Rarely is identity ever fixed in neat categories. Look at the example of the Native American Freedmen. Early in the 1800s, some Black Africans were enslaved by Native American groups in the south such as the Cherokee, or had escaped slavery and joined other groups, such as the Seminole. During the movement west with the Trail of Tears, these Black Africans traveled with the Native tribes on the Trail of Tears to places such as Oklahoma. After the Civil War and emancipation, the citizenship of these groups came under scrutiny and has been contested ever since.

> **Resources**
> Healy, J. (2020, September 8). Black, Native American and fighting for recognition in Indian Country. *The New York Times*.
> https://www.nytimes.com/2020/09/08/us/enslaved-people-native-americans-oklahoma.html.

> Film: *By Blood*. (2015). Marcos Barbery and Sam Russell. This film tells the story of the 'freedmen'—African Americans who trace their lineage to freed slaves who became members of various tribes, including the Seminole and Cherokee Nation. The Cherokee and Seminole Nations, 150 years later, now wealthy tribes with land, casinos and business holdings, continue to deny tribal rights to Freedmen descendants arguing that they are not members of their tribe 'by blood'.
> See the below articles for updates on the controversies relating to the Freedmen:
> Healy, J. (2020, September 8). Black, Native American and fighting for recognition in Indian Country. *The New York Times*. https://www.nytimes.com/2020/09/08/us/enslaved-people-native-americans-oklahoma.html.
> Walker, M. (2021, February 24). Cherokee Nation addresses bias against descendents of enslaved people. *The New York Times*. https://www.nytimes.com/2021/02/24/us/politics/cherokee-nation-black-freedmen.html.

Currently, most of the data available about the Indigenous population in the U.S. are limited to the categories of American Indian and Alaska Native (AI/AN). Sometimes Native Hawaiian and Pacific Islanders are put into a category together, and sometimes those groups are included within the Asian category. As we have already described, AI/AN refers to a person having origins in any of the original people of North or South America (including Central America) and who maintains tribal affiliation or community attachment (U.S. Office of Management and Budget, 1997). In the 2010 Census, 2,932,248 identified as AI/AN 'alone' and 5.2 million identified as AI/AN alone or 'in combination' with other race or ethnic identities. Racial or ethnic identity in the U.S. Census is self-selected, so anyone can choose to put anything they want on the census forms.

The Hispanic ethnicity category makes identity even more complicated as viewed through data sources such as the Census (see Cohn, 2010). Overall, our point here is that rarely does identity fall into neat categories of 'Black', 'White', 'Native American', or any other identity. While we have used racial and ethnic identity as examples in this section, we could just as well have discussed the complexities of other identities such as gender or sexualities, religion, or disabilities.

Revisiting Identity, Languages

In healthcare and human services work, we often are required to ask our clients their racial or ethnic identity. For culturally safe practice, it's important to consider how you ask these questions. Sometimes, it might be culturally safe to explain first why you are asking particular questions. If an individual's response could have resulted in a loss of rights, deemed illegal or immoral or any other imposed judgment experienced in the past, the seemingly harmless question asked by professionals today could trigger mistrust or anxiety for some people.

Throughout this book, we have talked about the complexity of the Indigenous populations and the terms used to describe them. Is 'Indigenous', as a category, adequate to understand the 'Indigenous' population in the U.S? Look at the map above of languages of Native America. There were originally hundreds of Indigenous languages in the U.S. with less than 200 Native languages spoken today. In California alone there have been 64 distinct languages (California Department of Parks and Recreation, n.d.). Each language group has its own culture—its own traditions, rituals, and beliefs. While there may be overlap, overall, what this shows us is that the 'Indigenous' population is diverse and has evolved over time. What you might learn or understand about people in New York, for example, may not necessarily apply to people in Chicago or Tulsa.

> **Reading**
> Hinton, L. (1994). *Flutes of fire: Essays on California Indian languages.* Berkeley, CA: Heyday Books.

There are over 350 different languages spoken in homes in the U.S. (U.S. Census, 2015) and what those languages are can be very different depending on what city you are looking at. For example, 38% of homes in the New York metro area speak a language other than English at home. In Los Angeles, it's 54% and around 15% in Philadelphia. Most cities have well over 100 different languages spoken at home. This diversity of languages, within and between cities and regions in the U.S., is just one example that illustrates the importance of 'keeping it local', which we discuss often throughout this book and is important to constantly keep in mind. How might knowing that there is so much language diversity in the U.S. and possibly in your local area influence how you practice in more culturally safe ways?

> **Reading**
> Below is the abstract from a paper that explored Appalachian identity. Geographic residence in the U.S. can be a strong aspect of identity such as for those who live in areas described as Appalachia. As with many identities, stigmas associated with this identity can influence self-identification and health and well-being.
>
> Krok-Schoen, J. L., Palmer-Wackerly, A. L., Dailey, P. M., & Krieger, J. L. (2015). The conceptualization of self-identity among residents of Appalachia Ohio. *Journal of Appalachian Studies, 21*(2), 229–246.
>
> Abstract: Social identity and its association to culture, place, and health is an important, but understudied, area of research. One social group that illustrates this connection between place and identity is people living in Appalachia. This exploratory mixed-method study investigates the appropriateness of the self-concept of Ohio Appalachian adults with cancer as 'Appalachian', the context associated with that identity and its association with community identification, rural identity, Appalachian Regional Commission (ARC) status, demographic data, and clinical trial (CT) enrollment. Forty-nine adults with cancer residing in Appalachia were recruited. Participants were cancer patients who (1) were offered a randomized clinical cancer trial; and (2) lived in or were treated in one of the thirty-two rural Appalachian counties in Ohio. Forty-seven percent of participants identified themselves as Appalachian and were reluctant to self-identify as Appalachian because of negative stereotypes or uncertainty about the term. Furthermore, many participants endorsed their residence within Appalachia but not their own identity. Future studies should

> utilize a culturally grounded approach and community-based methodology to explore how residents of Appalachian communities define their community and self-identification in order to improve health in the region.

> **Making It Local**
> - How are various population groups in your area presented in the media?
> - Are there different media outlets for different groups or communities? For example, are there newspapers, radio stations, or Facebook groups for specific groups in your area?
>
> In addition to statistics, maps, health data and information, television, news, movies, and literature can all provide ways for us to increase our awareness and sensitivity to cultural differences. What can you find for other groups within your community?

Conclusion

In this chapter we provided a wide range of data and information to think about when learning about health in the U.S. It is important to be careful interpreting statistics which, while useful, must be examined in conjunction with other sources of 'evidence'. Population structures, demographic mapping, languages, and other data show some stark differences that should be considered when setting up and delivering health services. All of the statistics presented in this chapter relate to real people. While the numbers may be important for health and human services professionals, the lived experiences gives insights that the statistics cannot provide.

References

Agency for Healthcare Research and Quality. (2018). *The distribution of the U.S. primary care workforce.* Content last reviewed July 2018. Agency for Healthcare Research and Quality. https://www.ahrq.gov/researchfindings/factsheets/primary/pcwork3/index.html.

Arias, E. (2016). *Changes in life expectancy by race and Hispanic origin in the United States, 2013–2014* (NCHS data brief, no 244). National Center for Health Statistics. https://www.cdc.gov/nchs/products/databriefs/db244.htm.

California Department of Parks and Recreation. (n.d.). *California Indians language groups.* https://www.parks.ca.gov/?page_id=23548.

Cohn, D. (2010). *Census history: Counting Hispanics.* Pew Research Center: Social and Demographic Trends. https://www.pewsocialtrends.org/2010/03/03/census-history-counting-hispanics-2/.

Dewees, S., & Marks, B. (2017). *Twice invisible, understanding rural native America* (Research Note #2). First Nations Development Institute. https://www.usetinc.org/wp-content/uploads/bvenuti/WWS/2017/May%202017/May%208/Twice%20Invisible%20-%20Research%20Note.pdf.

Office of Management and Budget (OMB). (1997). *Standards on race and ethnicity.* https://www.census.gov/topics/population/race/about.html.

Schaeffer, K. (2019). *The most common age among Whites in the U.S. is 58: More than double that of racial and ethnic minorities.* https://www.pewresearch.org/fact-tank/2019/07/30/most-common-age-among-us-racial-ethnic-groups/.

U.S. Census Bureau. (2011). *Population distribution and change: 2000 to 2010.* https://www.census.gov/prod/cen2010/briefs/c2010br-01.pdf.

U.S. Census Bureau. (2012). *The American Indian and Alaska Native population: 2010.* 2010 Census Briefs. https://www.census.gov/history/pdf/c2010br-10.pdf.

U.S. Census Bureau. (2015). *Census Bureau reports at least 350 languages in U.S. homes.* https://www.census.gov/newsroom/press-releases/2015/cb15-185.html.

U.S. Census Bureau. (2020). *Annual estimates of the resident population by sex, age, race alone or in combination, and Hispanic origin for the United States: April 1, 2010 to July 1, 2019* (NC-EST2019-ASR5H).

9

Special Interest and Priority Areas

In this chapter, *Special Interest and Priority Areas,* we explore areas that warrant special interest in the U.S., including maternal and child health, chronic and infectious disease, substance abuse, mental health, disability and aging. This chapter focuses on just some of the current major health issues faced in the U.S. and the potential role of professionals in addressing these in a culturally safe manner. It offers rationales for giving attention to certain groups and issues and asks readers to consider what issues are relevant in their local settings. It is not possible to look at all major health concerns, so we will review a selection of the key national priorities.

Chapter Objectives

After completing this chapter, you should be able to:

- identify some of the major health issues affecting our nation today
- describe leading health indicators and objectives that inform public health initiatives

- describe major health issues from a social determinants perspective
- identify cultural safety considerations among special interest and priority health concerns.

What Are Our Priorities?

For a book for use in health psychology and human services, how could we not cover topics such as diabetes, cardiovascular disease, or cancer? Aren't these the health issues and conditions that warrant our attention? Or should we discuss gun violence, militarism, police brutality, and incarceration? There are so many topics that we could cover, but our main goal is to show *how* cultural safety analysis and practice can be implemented through a small selection of topics.

Similarly, we could explore in more depth the health of various populations, such as the top concerning health issues among Black Americans, Indigenous Peoples, veterans, etc.… but, as discussed earlier in this book, we can't possibly learn everything we would need to know about any group. With a cultural safety approach, we need to look at ourselves and our own cultures and identities. We also know the potential to inadvertently stereotype groups and individuals that can do more harm than good. Having an understanding of various groups of people, at the same time, is critical for the effective and appropriate delivery of health and human services, as the previous chapter indicated.

We might know that overall, in the U.S., heart disease, cancers, and accidents are the top three leading causes of death. But these are not the same when you start to disaggregate the data by various variables, such as rural versus urban, race or ethnicity, sexuality, veteran status, disability, etc. So, if we were to completely base our resources for health priorities on these aggregate outcomes, some groups would be underserved as their own health priorities don't make the cut. What do we do, as professionals, when the priority, as we see it, does not align with those of clients in our care?

In the determinants of health chapter, we explored the social and economic contexts that lead to various health and social conditions and inequities. In this chapter, we consider some areas of special interest, keeping in mind that these health and social conditions are *produced* by the pervasive social and economic conditions. That is, put another way, they are *symptoms* of systematic oppression, the inequitable distribution of resources and power, and structural discrimination.

Statistically speaking, professionals will work with a diversity of clients regardless of intent or preferences. The fact that we have the health concerns that we do, within a very wealthy nation, should be cause for greater attention from health and human service professions. Health is not only the domain of health and human service workforces. In the determinants of health chapter, we identified the need for a more cohesive and collaborative approach to health and well-being that spans disciplines and sectors such as education, housing, employment, and justice.

Despite being one of the wealthiest nations in the world, the U.S. experiences some very poor health outcomes. These health concerns impact some populations and communities disproportionately. While it would be easier to attribute these health disparities to biological or behavioral differences, there is ample evidence to refute such simple explanations.

> **Critical Thinking**
> - What are the current health priorities in your state or region? Are there differing health priorities for different population groups? What might be some of the factors contributing to these differing health priorities and outcomes?

Healthy People: U.S. Priorities

In 1979, Surgeon General Julius Richmond issued a report 'Healthy People: The Surgeon General's Report on Health Promotion and Disease Prevention', which began the *Healthy People* initiative. Every ten years since 1980, the U.S. Department of Health and Human Services develops and reports on health promotion and disease prevention goals and objectives. *Healthy People 2020* was launched in December of 2010, which included four overarching goals:

- Attain high-quality, longer lives free of preventable disease, disability, injury, and premature death.
- Achieve health equity, eliminate disparities, and improve the health of all groups.
- Create social and physical environments that promote good health for all; and
- Promote quality of life, healthy development, and healthy behaviors across all life stages.

Healthy People 2020 included 42 Topic Areas and 1,300 Objectives. These are further broken down into 12 Leading Health Indicators with 26 Objectives. Table 9.1 shows the objectives for each of the 12 Leading Health Indicators. For example, Environmental Quality is measured through the objectives of an Air Quality Index greater than 100 and reducing the numbers of children exposed to secondhand smoke. In 2017, *The Midcourse Review* report was released which provides data and information on the progress toward the *Healthy People 2020* goals and objectives.

The learnings from *Healthy People 2020* informed the new initiative, *Healthy People 2030*. The Framework of *Healthy People 2030* includes a Vision, Mission, Foundational Principles, Overarching Goals and a Plan of Action. The number of objectives has been reduced with objectives falling into topic areas that include health conditions, health behaviors, populations, settings and systems, and the social determinants of health. Importantly, for the first time, *Healthy People 2030* will also include personal and organizational health literacy.

The criteria for the Leading Health Indicators for *Healthy People 2030* will:

- Focus on upstream measures, like risk factors and behaviors, instead of disease outcomes (remember the story of the river of health we discussed earlier)
- Address issues of national importance

Table 9.1 *Healthy People 2020* leading health indicators and objectives

Leading Health Indicators	Objectives
Access to health services	Persons with medical insurance
	Persons with a usual primary care provider
Clinical preventive services	Adults receiving colorectal cancer screening based on the most recent guidelines
	Adults with hypertension whose blood pressure is under control
	Persons with diagnosed diabetes whose A1c value is greater than 9%
	Children receiving the recommended vaccines
Environmental quality	Air Quality Index > 100
	Children exposed to secondhand smoke
Injury and violence	Injury deaths
	Homicides
Maternal, infant, and child health	All infant deaths
	Total preterm live births
Mental health	Suicide
	Adolescents with major depression
Nutrition physical activity and obesity	Adults meeting aerobic physical activity and muscle-strengthening objectives
	Obesity among adults
	Obesity among children and adolescents
	Mean daily intake of total vegetables
Oral health	Children, adolescents and adults who visited the dentist in the past year
Reproductive and sexual health	Sexually active females receiving reproductive health services
	Knowledge of serostatus among HIV-positive persons
Social determinants	Students graduating from high school 4 years after starting 9th grade

(continued)

Table 9.1 (continued)

Leading Health Indicators	Objectives
Substance abuse	Adolescents using alcohol or illicit drugs in the past 30 days
Tobacco	Adult cigarette smoking
	Adolescent cigarette smoking in the past 30 days

- Address high-priority public health issues
- Be modifiable in the short-term (through evidence-based interventions and strategies to motivate action at the national, state, local, and community levels)
- Address social determinants of health, health disparities, and health equity

> **Critical Thinking**
> - What looks different in *Healthy People 2030* compared with *Healthy People 2020*?
> - Recall the discussion in earlier chapters about evidence. How might this focus benefit some while disadvantaging others?
> - What ways could the issues of 'national importance' or 'high priority public health issues' become inequitable? Can you think of ways that these can be culturally safe and inclusive so as to not inadvertently lead to further inequalities?

> *Health disparities* are differences that exist among specific population groups in the U.S. in the attainment of full health potential that can be measured by differences in incidence, prevalence, mortality, burden of disease, and other adverse health conditions (NIH, 2014). Health disparities can stem from health inequities—systematic differences in the health

of groups and communities occupying unequal positions in society that are avoidable and unjust (Graham, 2004).

> **Activity**
> Find definitions for the following terms: morbidity, mortality, epidemic, pandemic, incidence, prevalence, burden of disease, or disease burden. Give an example for each term from national data sources.

Chronic Diseases

Chronic diseases are a national priority for everyone in the U.S. However, the predisposing factors and approaches for managing various health problems need to be put into context. Management and prevention approaches that may work for some people do not always work for everyone when the specific needs of individuals, groups, communities and their unique contexts are disregarded.

The major chronic diseases in the U.S. include diabetes, arthritis, cancer, epilepsy, heart disease, and stroke. It is believed that by targeting maternal health, there can be significant improvement in infant birth weight. This is underpinned by three main determinants: maternal and childhood education, the alleviation of poverty, and promoting a 'sense of control' and mental well-being.

> **Reading**
> For a comprehensive overview of the current state of chronic diseases, review the following reading.
> National Center for Chronic Disease Prevention and Health Promotion.

> https://www.cdc.gov/chronicdisease/resources/infographic/chronic-diseases.htm.

Chronic diseases have sometimes been referred to as 'lifestyle diseases', implying that the person with the chronic disease knowingly engaged in risk-taking behaviors that contributed to the development of the disease. This way of thinking emerges from biomedical and behavioral views of health that pay little attention to the socio-environmental and historical factors implicated in chronic disease profiles.

The discourse (or the ways we talk about) of chronic illness often shows the underlying attitudes and assumptions about causes and responses. 'Lifestyle diseases' implies blame or a conscious choice on the part of the client. For many health professionals, the view that 'They just need to be educated...' is repeated with frequency throughout healthcare settings. Education is undoubtedly a powerful contributor to enhancing health outcomes. However, the question might also be asked, 'Who else needs to be "educated"'?

Suggesting that chronic diseases such as diabetes or renal failure are *lifestyle* in origin denies the role of colonization in creating the environments that produce these health issues and in transforming lives to predispose people to such health problems. Colonization, like culture, is broadly defined here. Any one or group who are oppressed or disempowered can experience what it is to be 'colonized' by a more powerful group. Certainly, there are aspects within the control of individuals to manage or change and we are not suggesting that simply an awareness of our colonizing history is sufficient to change the outcomes toward better health. But it is important for professionals to examine their own beliefs about *why* people are at risk, in order to provide a relevant and meaningful support within their practice. For example, a belief statement about why someone might have a specific illness from a health professional's perspective may go:

You have chronic heart disease, because...

a. you don't exercise.

b. you don't understand the link between diet and ill-health.
c. you don't comply with your preventative treatments.
d. you don't care about your health.

A belief statement about why someone has chronic heart disease from another person's perspective may, depending on context and worldview, go something like:

I have chronic heart disease because…

a. It's a punishment for something I've done.
b. It's fate.
c. I live in a bad neighborhood.
d. I didn't believe I needed medication, because I felt OK.

Clients often have their own explanation of their problem or situation, and it may not match yours. Rather than try to convince or 'educate' the client about your beliefs, the client's explanations should be explored so that realistic solutions might be sought collaboratively. People of course may not offer a cultural or personal explanation, if a trust relationship hasn't first been established. Hopefully, through the preceding chapters, it has become abundantly clear that poor health today is not 'caused' by being whatever identity someone is. It is caused by a myriad of contextual influences; personal behavior is only one element of many.

This awareness requires professionals to monitor their responses in regard to clients, to avoid 'blaming the victim' and placing unrealistic and unworkable expectations on people who may have all the desire to become and stay healthy, but less of the control and opportunity. For many children born today, the reality is that a predisposition to chronic diseases starts in utero. Chronic diseases are much more prevalent in conditions of poverty, unemployment, and poor-quality education and housing. Health and human service professionals need to be alert to the possible co-morbidities and the implications this has for care.

Western approaches to chronic disease can tend to compartmentalize diseases and management. There is a focus on diabetes that is often separate from a focus on skin infections, which is often separate from a focus on cardiovascular disease, which is separate again from renal failure, and so on. However, providing holistic care is not simply a nice idea, it is good practice.

Infectious and Parasitic Diseases

Infectious diseases are illnesses that can be spread from one person to another that are caused by organisms like viruses and bacteria. The COVID-19 pandemic has demonstrated clearly that such a virus does not discriminate, but disparities among specific populations can increase risk. Other infectious diseases include HIV/Aids and other sexually transmitted diseases (STDs), the flu (influenza), tuberculosis (TB), and hepatitis.

When HIV first emerged in the U.S. we saw people vilified and discriminated against not only within public spaces, but within the very healthcare settings intended to provide care. People were labelled by the way they acquired HIV which can be sexually transmitted or through blood transfusions. Those that acquired the disease through blood tranfsusions were treated with empathy and compassion while those who acquired HIV through so-called 'lifestyle choices' were demeaned and subject to victim-blaming. The movie *Philadelphia* depicted a little of the discrimination faced by people affected by HIV.

Infectious disease rates have decreased dramatically within mainstream populations. Poverty, environmental conditions and lifestyle changes, however, have seen infectious disease rates rise. Many of the issues still being confronted in some regions relate to the lack of appropriate infrastructure and resources to maintain public health. This was demonstrated particularly clearly with the COVID-19 pandemic.

Think about what pre-public health New York or Los Angeles must have been like. What happened to garbage and water supply before the introduction of sanitation and garbage disposal services? While precontact lifestyles would have been less hazardous for Indigenous populations in terms of potential for infection, contemporary lifestyles are fraught with risks that require adequate education and resources to manage.

> **Reflection**
> Read this: '91,757 deaths from diseases of the heart, 84,443 from cancer, 28,831 from chronic lower respiratory diseases, 16,973 from cerebrovascular diseases (stroke), and 36,836 from unintentional injuries *potentially could be prevented each year*' (Yoon et al., 2014, emphasis added).
>
> What might your role as a professional be in effecting a change to this information? How could these deaths be prevented? It is all very well to advise people about health, hygiene, nutrition, and exercise but if the facilities and infrastructure are not present or not functioning, there is little value in the advice. Often, health and human service professionals, depending upon their disciplinary area, do not have an adequate picture of the home environment to be able to provide realistic advice. It is important therefore to get to know the communities with which you work. Establish positive relationships that allow you to work outside the clinical or community health centers and really get to know your clients' contexts in a way that is not reminiscent of the 'surveillance and intrusive' approaches of the past.

Handwashing is one simple but effective strategy to reduce the risk of infectious diseases. Although health professionals may often think this message should be well entrenched and understood, look at the number of hospital-related infections that are linked to less than adequate handwashing practices among health professionals.

What are parasitic diseases? 'The major neglected parasitic infections in the U.S. include Chagas disease, cysticercosis, toxocariasis, toxoplasmosis, and trichomoniasis. These five parasitic infections are considered "neglected" based on their high prevalence, chronic and disabling features, and their strong links with poverty' (Hotez, 2014). Of these 'neglected' infections, cysticercosis (tapeworm), toxocariasis (worms), and toxoplasmosis (parasite) can all be prevented by washing hands. But teaching people that washing their hands will have health benefits doesn't usually result in people washing their hands more!

At the start of the COVID-19 pandemic in early 2020, mass attempts were made to influence handwashing through social media, news, and throughout businesses and organizations around the world. Hand sanitizing stations were installed at entrances to stores, businesses and restaurants and throughout schools. Research found significant increases in handwashing behaviors from October 2019 to June of 2020, during the COVID-19 pandemic, with particular increases in handwashing after coughing, sneezing, or blowing the nose (Haston et al., 2020). Interestingly, those most unlikely to wash their hands were White adults, men, and young adults aged 18–24, suggesting the need to target handwashing to those groups.

> **Website**
> See the Global Handwashing Partnership website for some interesting information and resources: https://globalhandwashing.org/.

Infant and Maternal Health

For the wealthiest country in the world, one might expect various health statistics in the U.S. to be among the best, yet our infant mortality doesn't even rank in the top 50 countries. The U.S. ranks at only 55 globally with a rate of 5.80 deaths per 1,000 live births (CIA, World FactBook, 2017 data). Infant mortality varies substantially by state and by race and ethnicity in the U.S.

These infant mortality rates are certainly unacceptable within such a wealthy nation. While some improvements have occurred, the rates of morbidity have increased for those who do survive beyond the first year of life. Most children today have a better chance of survival at birth, but many will suffer greater levels of illness that are largely preventable. There are a number of national programs targeting infant and maternal health. Increasing access to antenatal services, and initiatives such as home visitations from childcare nurses, are a few strategies aimed at reducing disparities in this area.

Maternal health has been identified as possibly the most significant factor in the health of whole families. Family structures and child rearing practices are culturally determined. From a cultural safety perspective, it is important that health and human services professionals examine their preexisting views of what maternal roles and responsibilities should be, to enable culturally safe engagement with families.

> **Activity**
> - Find out how services in your region access the most vulnerable women and infants. What programs are available to this group?
> - Conduct a review of the literature to examine the responses of various states to infant and maternal health. What are the local policies and priorities?
> - What does the research say about health and social outcomes for families when health education is provided to mothers? Look globally as well.

Risky and High-Risk Substance Use

Risk behaviors are another area to consider when thinking about the range of factors contributing to the health disparities between groups. This area, however, can be somewhat contentious because people's behaviors are often believed to be within the *complete* power and control of the person engaging in those behaviors. For example, some people might say that the reason someone smokes cigarettes is 'because they want to'. But human behavior, as already discussed, is influenced by a range of factors. It is overly simplistic to suggest that someone engages in certain behaviors 'by choice' or 'because they want to'. It discounts other factors, including social conditions (such as friends and family), cultural, financial, environmental (e.g., not exercising because a neighborhood is not safe or conducive to exercise), and historical factors. Overall, information about health-risk behaviors needs to be considered within this broader context. Correspondingly, interventions need to be developed and delivered that take these wider contextual details into consideration.

Some of the health-risk behaviors that are disparate between groups include smoking and drinking alcohol at risky levels. There is no doubt that one of the most destructive influences to affect so many Americans has been substances of addiction.

> **Readings**
> National Institute on Alcohol Abuse and Alcoholism, Alcohol Facts and Statistics. https://www.niaaa.nih.gov/publications/brochures-and-fact-sheets/alcohol-facts-and-statistics.
> Moody, L., Satterwhite, E., & Bickel, W. K. (2017). Substance use in rural central Appalachia: Current status and treatment considerations. *Rural Mental Health, 41*(2), 123–135. https://doi.org/10.1037/rmh0000064. https://www.ncbi.nlm.nih.gov/pmc/articles/PMC5648074/.

> **Scenario**
> Kelly is a social worker for a home hospice care agency. Two years ago, her 19-year-old son died suddenly after a long battle with mental illness. She was consumed with guilt over his death and distraught that she should have been able to prevent his death. She was prescribed opioids by her family doctor for back pain related to heavy lifting at work. She started taking more of them because they helped calm her and she wouldn't think as much about her son's death. But she needed more and more to cope. She made some friends who could help her get heroin, and spiraled even further into dysfunction. She was struggling to take care of her other younger children and her marriage was falling apart. Every day the goal was to figure out how to get the money and the drugs to get her through the day. She went to a drug rehab, promising herself and her family that she would do better. But it was already too late. Kelly had contracted an infection from using dirty needles. She refused the needed intravenous antibiotics and hospitalization and died. She was just 46 years old.
> - Where were the points of intervention that may have avoided this outcome?

> - How might Kelly's cultural identity have contributed to a lack of support from services, i.e., a college-educated, health professional, married with children.
> - How did Kelly's issues go undetected for so long?
> - How might it have helped to have family involved in health appointments or assessments?
> - What role did the friends play in Kelly's outcome?
> - Why might Kelly have refused treatment in the end?
> - Have you made any previously unexamined assumptions about Kelly in terms of her social class, ethnicity, or character?
> - Did you think that Kelly's story started with her son's issues—and possibly even further back? People can be high functioning and falling apart at the same time. Some health professionals overlook family input, concerned about their patient's confidentiality, but it is often valuable to encourage patients to bring a support person who they are happy to have with them.

Opioid Epidemic in the U.S.

The opioid epidemic in the U.S. is one example of how our medical system can gradually cause harm. While opioids are incredibly useful for patients in extreme pain, their use (and misuse) created a national crisis that hit its peak in 2017 with 47,600 deaths involving any opioid. Opioids are highly addictive.

One of the large pharmaceutical companies that makes OxyContin, an opioid that was an early driver of the opioid epidemic, has been involved in lawsuits and pled guity to criminal wrongdoing for aggressively marketing opioids. As a result, they have paid billions of dollars toward drug treatment and dealing with other effects of the opioid epidemic.

Asking clients about changing behaviors such as quitting smoking, or quitting drinking, can sometimes seem like a pointless or unwelcome exercise, but it can be helpful to remember that people trying to break an addiction often make several attempts before they are successful. Even if a client seems disinterested or unappreciative of the conversation, don't give up on raising the issue. This might be the one time that they are ready to go.

> **Making It Local**
> Review the newspapers and other media for issues relating to alcohol and drug use among various population groups? What is the nature of the items presented?
> How balanced is the representation? What drug and alcohol programs are available in your region?
> Look up your local chapters of 12-step recovery meetings such as Alcoholics Anonymous or Narcotics Anonymous. How many meetings are held in your area? These 12-step recovery meetings have Open meetings, which are open for anyone to attend who has an interest. As a health or human service professional, chances are, you will have clients (or friends and family, or even yourself) who are in recovery or who would benefit from attending 12-step recovery meetings. Attending an open meeting, whether or not you identify as an addict or alcoholic, can be very valuable in your work with your clients. Search for an open meeting in your area and attend. Introduce yourself to someone when you get there and let them know that you are there to observe. If someone calls on you to talk, you can introduce yourself as an observer and pass on talking. Make sure to connect with people after the meeting.

Mental Health and Social and Emotional Well-Being

Mental health issues, like other health issues, are embedded in a larger set of questions relating to culture and cultural differences, historical events, social and cultural change and coping. Who defines mental health and ill-health and whose worldview is used to do this are important considerations. For example, how would you respond if a client told you they knew of a man who was hung on a cross and came back from the dead three days later? If you were familiar with Christian ideas about the resurrection of Jesus, you would probably accept this as being part of the person's belief system and not even think about calling for mental health assessment. If another person told you that the reason they were sick was due to snakes in their chest, how would you respond? Does it depend upon your worldview?

Paying attention to differing worldviews is a relatively recent phenomenon in health, and some disciplines are more attentive than others. There is a growing body of literature focusing on the challenges of cross-cultural mental health assessment and counseling. An important consideration of cross-cultural mental health assessment is being able to ascertain whether someone's behaviors, thoughts or expressions are appropriate within their cultural context or not.

> **Scenario**
> Read the following example of culturally unsafe mental health assessment that had a disastrous impact for the individual concerned:
>
>> ...Rita Quintero, a Mexican native who was found wandering the streets of a Kansas town. She seemed to be dressed oddly, seemed not to have bathed recently, and was not able to communicate except for a few Spanish words. She was involuntarily committed and remained hospitalized for 12 years. During her commitment she was treated against her will with psychotropic drugs. It was eventually determined that she was a member of the Tarahumara Indian tribe of Mexico. Her appearance, dress, and behaviors, which had been described as odd and indicative of mental illness, were actually traditional aspects of her culture. She had only a limited grasp of Spanish because she was a native speaker of Ramuri, a tribal language. After a Ramuri interpreter was located, she was released and allowed to return to her home.
>
> - What strategies could have been employed to ensure this person's cultural, psychological, and physical safety?
> - What does the experience suggest about the preparation of professionals to work in a culturally safe way?
>
> This case study is presented in a cultural competence resource, *Quintero v. Encarnacion*. https://aspph-wp-production.s3.us-east-1.amazonaws.com/app/uploads/2014/04/11-278-CulturCompet-Interactive-final.pdf.

> **Resources**
> *Mad In America* is a fabulous website with lots of resources relevant to mental health and well-being. The website includes blogs, videos, continuing education programs, current news, and research. https://www.madinamerica.com/.
>
> Snyder, S. N., Pitt, K., Shanouda, F., Voronka, J., Reid, J., & Landry, D. (2019). Unlearning through Mad Studies: Disruptive pedagogical praxis. *Curriculum Inquiry, 49*(4), 485–502. https://doi.org/10.1080/03626784.2019.1664254.
> https://www.tandfonline.com/doi/abs/10.1080/03626784.2019.1664254?journalCode=rcui20.

> **Making It Local**
> - How do people think about mental health and illness in your area? What about within your family—are there any strongly expressed views about mental health issues?
> - How would you determine your client's and their family's cultural understandings of mental health and illness?
> - In your opinion, how important is it for your clients to understand the Western medical explanation of mental illness?
> - From your own professional standpoint (e.g., nurse, doctor, social worker, psychologist), what are the important facts about mental illness (as understood by Western medicine) that would need to be communicated to families?

As students and future professionals, it is essential that you conduct your own analyses of what is presented to you about health and well-being and the variations among different populations and groups. Actively interrogate how reports and other sources are presenting information about groups and populations. Reflect on how materials might cause further harm by contributing to stigma and stereotypes that perpetuate harm.

When confronted with information that shows disparities between groups, always ask what created these situations? How did it come to be this way? Health and human service professionals can continue to treat the symptoms, but they also need to consider the causes. Causes, as we learned in the chapter about the social determinants of health, are complicated and rarely simple. Causes can be like the layers of an onion. Once you pull back one layer, there is another beneath it. Keep pulling back the layers and embrace the complexity and resist the urge to reduce causes to simplistic or singular events.

Aging

We learned earlier that Indigenous, Black, and Hispanic populations may be younger in terms of demographic profiling, but diseases and other health problems related to aging are experienced much earlier than in White and Asian populations. The different population profiles may at least partially explain why so little attention has been given to the issues of aging for many in the U.S. It is increasingly apparent that the costs—personal, social, and economic—are substantial.

Furthermore, given the acute and chronic disease profiles, the diseases normally associated with aging are experienced much earlier. Students and professionals are often shocked to encounter people in their thirties and forties in the hospital and community health systems with chronic lung disease, cognitive impairments, as well as cardiac, renal and a range of other health issues normally associated with people in their sixties and beyond.

What makes for a positive aging experience can be subjective, but it can, like most aspects of health, also be culturally determined. Think about your own picture of healthy aging. For some readers, that may be a distant picture, for others it may be quite close. For many cultural and racial groups globally, there is generally a strong reverence for the elders of society who are viewed as holders of knowledge, experience, and authority. Physical indicators of aging in some cultures, far from being perceived negatively, can be valued. Think about your own cultural values toward grey or white hair, for example. The signs of the first grey hairs in the authors' cultures are often met with trips to the hairdresser to cover up an obvious indicator of aging. Yet, in other cultures, it is when someone has grey or white hair that they are really regarded with respect and authority. Recent years have seen trends in young people intentionally coloring their hair grey, silver, or white.

While traditional values may place great importance on the elderly in society, today there are considerable pressures impacting on communities generally, which can result in a loss of respect and valuing of the elderly. What might this mean in contexts where the role of the elderly is so crucial? Think about the impact of losing significant sections of a society prematurely. Statistically speaking, many groups are likely to die earlier than White or Asian Americans. For those who do attain what is considered old age, it is important to think about what a culturally safe, healthy aging might be. How will you judge this as a practitioner?

> **Reading**
> National Institute on Aging. (n.d.). The National Institute on Aging: Strategic Directions for Research, 2020–2025, Goal F: Understand health disparities related to aging and develop strategies to improve the health status of older adults in diverse populations. Accessed from: https://www.nia.nih.gov/about/aging-strategic-directions-research/goal-health-disparities-adults.

Assessments

Whether for pain, cognitive, or other issues, there is a need to evaluate the validity of health assessment tools for the diversity of clients who may require care. Assessment tools made for a particular cultural group may not be appropriate for assessing the needs of someone from outside of the target group.

From a cultural safety perspective, this is critical to ensuring that care is determined on the basis of screenings and assessments that do not have a cultural bias to them. Please note this is referring to tools of assessment, such as pain scores that use faces or numbers. Remember the reference earlier to the academic text that published stereotyped views of pain behaviors based on ethnicity. There is no cultural group that does not experience pain but assessing people's pain behaviors based on preconceived ideas is not only culturally unsafe, it's clinically unsafe, leading some to be under or over medicated and not be listened to in response to their experience of pain.

Ouldred (2004) points out the cultural bias that renders most standardized tests ineffective or inappropriate for use with people of differing cultural backgrounds. That is, people from non-Western cultures may have difficulty with some of the concepts and words used in the tests. A lower score may be misinterpreted to indicate cognitive impairment (or depression, depending on the test), but is actually only reflecting cultural misunderstanding or lack of exposure to culturally dependent concepts.

> **Activity**
> - Have a look at various assessment tools available for pain, cognitive, or other assessments. Reflect on their usefulness for intercultural assessment. Who has been involved in their development?
> - Can you see any cultural bias in the tools?
> - Can you find tools developed for specific cultural groups?
> - What might be the consequences of using culturally biased or inappropriate tools?

(Dis)abilities

Disability is often measured by considering the limitations of a person to perform their daily core activities. Profound or severe core activity limitation means that a person always or sometimes needs help with at least one core activity of daily living. Core activities of daily living include eating, sleeping, and hygiene. Disabilities can be any impairment that prevents someone from easily participating in an activity such as walking, talking, seeing, hearing, thinking, etc. Disabilities are not deficits. Some language groups don't even have words for disabilities suggesting an inclusivity rather than othering.

Overall, attitudes toward people with disabilities have changed over time with increased awareness, support, and systemic and structural changes that make society more inclusive and accessible for people with diverse abilities. Think about how buildings and spaces are or are not accessible for various abilities. Even though we have policies against discrimination toward people with various abilities, it would not be difficult to find examples of stigmatizing and exclusion that continue today.

An important cultural safety consideration here is to examine your own possible biases and assumptions regarding abilities. The idea that everyone with a disability will necessarily want to 'fix' their particular issue if they could, has the potential to diminish someone who does not see their disability as problematic.

> **Critical Thinking**
> - How would you respond to a client who refused a cochlear implant that might allow them to hear? What if the decision was being made for a child?
> - By insisting that such a choice would improve their quality of life, what message are you giving about how you perceive the individual?
> - How would you engage in such a conversation in a culturally safe way?

Social media has provided increased virtual support for people with a variety of abilities such that people no longer need to be in close geographic proximity to get support in community with others sharing similar experiences.

Hearing loss is a health issue that has far reaching impacts. With around 1 in 7 people experiencing some level of hearing loss, it's certainly important to be aware of the possibility of hearing loss and how it can affect individuals, their families, and extend into community. Hearing loss among young children can impact early language development, as well as relationships and behavior. Educational experiences and opportunities can be significantly impacted among school-aged children with hearing loss. As hearing loss increases with age, family relationships can become strained and people experiencing hearing loss may become increasingly isolated. For those who experience complete hearing loss, inclusion in family and social life is facilitated by the existence of hand language or signing but for some, hearing impairment added to other physical challenges can lead to social exclusion and isolation for the elderly, along with diminished roles and responsibilities.

Reading
Clare, E. (2017). *Brilliant imperfection: Grappling with cure.* Duke University Press.

Poem
Taking account of all the various health issues discussed in this chapter, read the following poem while keeping in mind our interactions with so many people as health and human services providers and how our care processes and interactions can inadvertently dehumanize the very people we aim to help.

She Hate Her Body, by Whisper Young
> She hate her body
> But she can't tell nobody
> 'Cause other's eyes don't believe their ears even after they've seen what she say
> For this they press fingers to her lips
> Denying her thighs and hips
> So she hate her body
> With all its smears and smudges
> From all those touches
> See she's tried bleaches and accents
> But none of them be erasin' the stench
> Of all those hand and eye prints
> And she hate they smell
> So she hate her shell
> She hate her body
> 'Cause it's called her's but it don't belong to her

It belongs to the others
With their stares and uninvited...touches
So she prays and waits for heaven
As she play invisible as hell
Swallowing her tongue so her lips won't tell
What her soul yelllllll
That she hate to breathe so free
And speak so full and loud
That she hate being denied yet passed around
That she hate her crown
It's too easy to grip for those attempting to pull her down
So she covers that shit to blend in
To blend in and be loved
'Cause her body want things it has needs
Needs that leave her cursed when she heeds them
But they call her worse when she don't meet them
She hate this body because everyone but her is allowed to decide where it goes, what it does, what it needs
Yet they deny her screams
They even deny her bandages when it bleeds
It's her's, her's, her's but they've confiscated it
They possess it for hatred and pleasure
So caught in their label making, boxing, shipping, pattern clipping while unique fabric stripping
That no one sees.....her
So she hate her body
And every day when she looks in the mirror she attempts to make up where she falls short till she hate her
And NOTHING can make her see invisible beauty
Trapped in bodies....who hate....themselves

Critical Thinking

- In what ways can healthcare and human services work lead to someone feeling like their body is not their own? What other reasons might the writer be alluding to for feeling their body was not their own?
- What actual legislation can you find in which the government dictates control of people's bodies?
- Can you come up with examples of how healthcare and human services work can lead to someone feeling like they cannot speak up to ask for what they need or if they do not agree with something?
- How can professional work do better? Can you come up with some examples?

Conclusion

This chapter examined only a few of the numerous health issues of concern in the U.S. Many of you will have areas of interest that you will hopefully pursue independently. Other topics such as gender and health, growth and nutrition, palliative care, and so on, could all just as easily have been discussed. However, as professionals, the onus is very much on you to seek out the information and learning necessary to make your professional practice culturally safe in any setting.

References

American Public Health Association. (n.d.). *Disparities in the U.S.* https://www.apha.org/what-is-public-health/generation-public-health/disparities-in-the-us.

American Public Health Association. (n.d.). *Racism and health.* https://www.apha.org/topics-and-issues/health-equity/racism-and-health.

Baciu, A., Negussie, Y., Geller, A., et al. (Eds.). (2017). *The state of health disparities in the U.S.* National Academies of Sciences, Engineering, and Medicine; Health and Medicine Division; Board on Population Health and Public Health Practice; Committee on Community-Based Solutions to Promote Health Equity in the United States. National Academies Press (US). https://www.ncbi.nlm.nih.gov/books/NBK425844/.

Graham, H. (2004). Social determinants and their unequal distribution: Clarifying policy understandings. *Milbank Quarterly, 82*(1), 101–124.

Hotez, P. J. (2014). Neglected parasitic infections and poverty in the United States. *PLoS Neglected Tropical Diseases, 8*(9), e3012. https://doi.org/10.1371/journal.pntd.0003012.

Haston, J. C., Miller, G. F., Berendes, D., et al. (2020). Characteristics associated with adults remembering to wash hands in multiple situations before and during the COVID-19 pandemic—United States, October 2019 and June 2020. *MMWR Morbidity and Mortality Weekly Report, 69,* 1443–1449. http://dx.doi.org/10.15585/mmwr.mm6940a2externalicon.

Healthy People 2030. (n.d.). *Social determinants of health.* U.S. Department of Health and Human Services, Office of Disease Prevention and

Health Promotion. https://health.gov/healthypeople/objectives-and-data/social-determinants-health.

NIH (National Institutes of Health). (2014). *Health disparities*, November 2, 2016. http://www.nhlbi.nih.gov/health/educational/healthdisp.

Ouldred, E. (2004). Screening for dementia in older people. *British Journal of Community Nursing, 9,* 434–437.

Yoon, P. W., Bastian, B., Anderson, R. N., Collins, J. L., & Jaffe, H. W. (2014). *Potentially preventable deaths from the five leading causes of death—United States, 2008–2010.* U.S. Center for Disease Control.

10

Capacity and Resilience

The tendency of health and human service professionals and governments to focus on the perceived deficits rather than on the strengths of various groups has been evident throughout America's history. A cultural safety approach requires a reorientation—from positioning certain populations as problematic to focusing on strengths, capacity and resilience. Such a reorientation also fits well with the principles of primary health care (PHC) and community psychology.

This chapter explores the potential for success in health and social outcomes that can be achieved from a simple change in view, while also maintaining the stance that improvement in the health of all sectors of the community is everyone's responsibility.

Chapter Objectives

After completing this chapter, you should be able to:

- define and critically analyze the concepts of capacity, resilience, cultural vitality, and strengths-based models

© The Author(s), under exclusive license to Springer Nature Switzerland AG 2021
P. B. Thompson and K. Taylor, *A Cultural Safety Approach to Health Psychology*, Sustainable Development Goals Series, https://doi.org/10.1007/978-3-030-76849-2_10

- examine the role of capacity and resilience in achieving improved health outcomes for all
- identify assumptions, beliefs, and attitudes that overlook or diminish capacity and resilience
- analyze the role of health and human service professionals in supporting individuals and groups' capacity and resilience.

Concepts: Capacity, Resilience, Cultural Vitality

While 'health' is often couched in terms of ill-health, injury, or disease, at the same time, many government departments, funding agencies, and organizations claim to focus on *building capacity* in communities when it comes to marginalized or vulnerable populations. Let's look at this terminology. What does this say to health professionals to talk about *building* capacity? It implies certain populations are without capacity or resilience and that this needs to be provided by those external bodies who are seemingly more 'capable'.

We are not suggesting that there is not a role for supporting or promoting capacity and resilience. But as with much already discussed, it is the way something is done that determines the cultural safety of an approach. Most programs and services in the U.S. today are developed and delivered by departments and organizations that may not be representative of the client groups. While it may be quicker and easier and likely cheaper for a 'remote bureaucrat' to develop a program or service that will then be delivered or 'rolled out' across the country—the inequalities between population groups suggest that this approach is not working. One of the reasons why this approach may not work is that the people who are affected by these programs and services (for example, as service users) have often not had any contribution to the development of those programs. Capacity building is partly about providing the opportunities and spaces for recipients of targeted programs to participate in, contribute to and manage programs and services for themselves.

Empowerment can be defined as a multilevel construct that involves people assuming control and mastery over their lives in the context of their social and political environment. It can also be described as a social action process that promotes participation of people, organizations, and communities toward the goals of increased individual and community control, political efficacy, improved quality of community life, and social justice (Wallerstein, 1992, p. 198). Empowerment may also mean handing over control to an outside organization, which can seem contradictory. If we look at the example of residential schools for Native Americans, children were forced to attend, the community was disempowered and divided, and many suffered ongoing trauma as a result. Today, however, it may well be an empowered act for families to choose to send their children to a boarding school as an option that other Americans might also make for their children. The key word is 'choose'. Cultural safety, as noted, is about not assuming what someone will or won't do on the basis of some preconceived idea or stereotype. It is about talking with people and decolonizing our approaches to ensure the client is empowered and, in a position, to make an informed choice.

Resilience is a concept that relates to the ability of some people to 'bounce back' from difficult situations. Resilience is positive adaptation despite significant adversity (Luthar, 2003). It is a concept that is often used in relation to children. The idea of finding out what makes some kids do well, even in high-risk environments such as abusive families or poverty, is that if we know what makes some people resilient, then we can use that to help others to be more resilient as well. 'Resilience is not a feature of children, but a process that involves interactions between attributes of children, their families, neighborhoods and wider social and cultural environments' (Lalonde, 2006, p. 54).

As with the concept of 'capacity', there are some critiques of the concept of resilience. The major critique is when resilience is thought of as a trait of certain people. It is important to remember that if we think of resilience as some *thing* inside certain people—that you either *have* it or you don't—then the usefulness of the concept is really questionable. What do we do to help people who are in difficult circumstances if they don't *have* resilience? We can then victim blame people for not being resilient enough.

One very helpful analogy of resilience is that of a tennis ball. If you throw a tennis ball against a wall, it bounces back. Life adversities are like the tennis ball being thrown against a wall. Resilience is the bouncing back. But if you were to video that tennis ball in slow motion to see what happens to it when it hits the wall, you would see that hitting the wall distorts the ball—adversity has effects, even if you cannot necessarily tell by looking at the ball later. But if you kept throwing that ball against the wall, over and over and over again, it would eventually stop bouncing back—it would lose its resilience. Or, you might think of a ball that never had a good bounce, a ball that maybe just wasn't 'resilient'. Much of the research focuses on the bounciness—the resilience—but some have argued that we should stop focusing so much on the resilience and, instead, stop throwing balls against the wall. That is, our focus should rather be on reducing adversity or causing distress, as discussed in the Determinants chapter.

Others suggest resilience can and should be taught. The response of people to COVID-19 has really tested the resilience of individuals and groups to adapt and move forward. We have had to adapt to new ways of working, new ways of engaging with others, and new ways of providing services. Resilience does not preclude us from experiencing certain emotions such as frustration, grief, or anger, but it does equip people to manage their responses in a healthy way. According to Dvorsky, et al. (2020):

> The coronavirus disease 2019 (COVID-19) pandemic presents tremendous challenges to child and adolescent health. It is expected that the COVID-19 crisis, including the disease and prolonged social distancing, will have a major impact on youth well-being… Schools are closed, businesses are shuttered, and families are adjusting to 24/7 interaction, while caregivers simultaneously navigate parenting, financial, and professional challenges and uncertainties…Risk is real and warrants attention. And yet a sole focus on risk will miss resilience processes that can advance science, services, education, and policy aimed at understanding how children and adolescents respond to crisis.

Masten (2001) cites research that shows:

> The study of resilience in development has overturned many negative assumptions and deficit-focused models about children growing up under

the threat of disadvantage and adversity. The most surprising conclusion emerging from studies of these children is the ordinariness of resilience… that resilience is common and that it usually arises from the normative functions of human adaptational systems, with the greatest threats to human development being those that compromise these protective systems.

Poem
Read the following poem from the perspective of what was just learned about capacity and resilience. Note: this poem contains language that some readers may find offensive.
Eyewitness, by Whisper Young

And the hood remains calm
Ain't no fear up in here
We see bullshit whether or not
  it's election year
We've come to accept it
There's no antiseptic
For our open wounds no matter
  who gets elected
Knowin' that the real
  muthafuckin'
Weapons of mass destruction
Look like soap chips
Make you run fast with someone
  else's merchandise in a tight grip
Sportin' seven coats and
  fashionably white lips
Yet the hood remains calm
Despite the sparks in the dark
Gettin' shot through the heart
Unafraid
Of Ak
Spray
Shots blown
You make sure our homes
Are in war zones

So our daughters and sons
Learn early on to duck and run
From guns
Only the hood die young, Homies
Just sometimes it's in them tired
  ass away jerseys
Oops 'scuse me please
I meant to say fatigues
The only things not camouflaged
  by the tan and or green
Are the words in black
On the back
That scream out MURDER ME
  PLEASE
Yet the hood remains calm
'Cause it was gonna happen
  anyway
Maybe in the park where the
  children play
Maybe in his doorway
While he was slowly reaching for
  his wallet
Maybe in the crack house, maybe
  in the project
So everything is solid
We ain't gettin' brolic
We been knew y'all gubment
  muhfukkas had some fucked up
  logic

So the hood remains calm
Without hesitation
Despite the frustration
We know the type of odds we facin'
That this shit right here ain't nothin' but a big ass plantation
Where you work our men to death
Then stand over them with a mason jar just collect their last breath
Take away right action
So we comprise less of the educated fraction
Become less of a faction
When we prosper, your only reaction
Is to pray and pray for our muhfukkin' destruction and downfall
But without us, who the hell y'all gone call
To build and make innovations for y'all
Bet I got you scared as Y2k now
'Cause if the darkies really left town
All your shit would shut the fuck down
Yet the hood remains calm
Watchin' the same television
You use to exploit our women
We not pretendin'
We don't see that shit
We're just immune to it
It don't botha us
We've developed a tolerance
You've been doin' the same shit since the beginning
Raping the sistahs in front of their men
Can't hear the screams or cries 'cause still
We do it by our own compromised will
And part of what makes us strong Goddesses
Is being their daughters, sisters, mothers, and lovers
So the hood remains calm
We defy
Despite your attempts to deny us
We remain survivors despite your attempts to ride us
And make us feel worthless
When you presented Ms. Berry with a gold statuette
The hood was not impressed
You shouldah been
Let our asses in
How about you get yo' ass in a time machine and do a backspin
Give a few to Ms. Mammy Johnson, a few to Ms. Dandridge, a few to Ms. Cicely Tyson
Then maybe my friends we could make amends
'Cause by the time Halle found Isaiah she should've already had about four or five of them
Been one of dem
Bond women
Before she was Queen she was a Goddess
Before she had a frolic
Even when we only seen her movies down in the projects
But to be honest
We recognize that
If her
Lips were a lil' thicker
Her skin wasn't lighter
And her nose was wider
You'd still love her less
Yet
The hood remains calm
Like Buddhist monks
With junk in the trunk, giving monster dunks, while eatin' free lunch with gold fronts

To protect our brothas from being killed
Despite the way that makes us all feel
Now we can't stand one anotha
Fed the bullshit that we must be liberated from our brothas
'Cause they're the only ones that choose to use and abuse us
So now between the sexes we have no trust
Runnin' a race to eliminate
Due to self hate
'Cause our brothas were made to care for, love and protect us

After all, y'all the ones that's really fucked up in the mind

Walking roun' blind
With no spines
It's more of us, plus we stay on the grind
We been facin' a war not waitin' for one to come
So we can run
And when it's all said and done

After all the bullshit you put on us to stop our lives
While we yet continue to reject demise
Who you think gone survive as the end approaches
Muhfukka us...and the cockroaches
So the hood remains calm...the hood remains calm...the hood remains calm

Critical Thinking

- What might the author of *Eyewitness* be talking about when she writes 'the hood remains calm'?
- What are some ways that resilience or courage are demonstrated?
- Did you notice the comparison she makes between gun violence in communities, team sports, and the military? What do these have in common?
- In what ways is the past interwoven with the present in this poem? How does that relate to our discussions of the impact of history and colonialism?

Cultural Vitality

Discussions of health can often distort the ways in which certain groups are perceived. While it may be a statistical reality that some populations live shorter and generally sicker lives, their capacity and strengths in adapting and responding to traumatic or challenging events are rarely examined. Furthermore, capacity and strength are rarely harnessed or identified by health and human services professionals as a valuable tool in addressing health inequities or in reorienting the thinking even further to promote health equity.

Cultural vitality has been defined as 'the emotional strength, the spirit, the essence of people who strive and struggle to maintain strong identity and adapt to new and challenging environments, while they value and pass on distinctive cultural beliefs, practices and life ways' (Eckermann et al., 2010, p. 99). In the concept of cultural vitality, the active and proactive adaptation of culture is assumed and valued, rather than 'culture' being seen as a static, idealized 'given' that needs to be 'gone back to'. This concept of cultural vitality suggests that health professionals need to consider the dynamic process of culture in relation to clients. Rather than focusing on the damage of colonization or the current 'problems' affecting communities, acknowledge and recognize the impact, but also acknowledge the innovative, creative and resourceful ways that people and their communities can, and have, responded.

Role of Health and Human Services Professionals

As we have mentioned frequently throughout this text, health and human services professionals are often in a position of power to influence clients in their care. That power can be used to facilitate empowerment and to build on resilience and accommodate capacity, rather than disempowering or focusing on deficits. In the clinical setting, it is easy for professionals to assume positions of great importance within communities and establish themselves as key to programs and activities linked to their service. However, the real achievement of any professional may be seen when programs and activities operate without their input. This is not to say that professionals have no role, but that the role is to promote self-reliance and capacity.

Readings

Below are a number of academic articles relating to capacity and resilience.

Teufel-Shone, N. I., Tippens, J. A., McCrary, H. C., Ehiri, J. E., & Sanderson, P. R. (2018). Resilience in American Indian and Alaska native public health: An underexplored framework. *American Journal of Health Promotion, 32*(2), 274–281. https://doi.org/10.1177/0890117116664708.

Hodge, F. S., Pasqua, A., Marquez, C.A., & Geishirt-Cantrell, B. (2002). Utilizing traditional storytelling to promote wellness in American Indian communities. *Journal of Transcultural Nursing, 13*(1), 6–11.

Struthers, R. (2003). The artistry and ability of traditional women healers. *Health Care Women International, 24*(4), 340–354.

Ungar, M. (2012). Researching and theorizing resilience across cultures and contexts. *Preventive Medicine, 55*(5), 387–389.

Ungar, M. (2011). The social ecology of resilience: Addressing contextual and cultural ambiguity of a nascent construct. *American Journal of Orthopsychiatry, 81*(1), 1–17.

Jurjonas, M., & Seekamp, E. (2018). Rural coastal community resilience: Assessing a framework in eastern North Carolina. *Ocean & Coastal Management, 162*, 137–150. ISSN 0964-5691. https://doi.org/10.1016/j.ocecoaman.2017.10.010.

The Jurjonas and Seekamp (2018) reading suggests that attributes of resilience should be considered in the development of health interventions. Attention to collective resilience is recommended to leverage existing assets in American Indian and Alaska Native communities.

Much of the literature from the health psychology domain focuses on stress and coping, trauma and trauma therapy. There are various schools of thought on these approaches and what is more or less beneficial. What would you find more helpful in dealing with a critical experience? There is a view that reinforcing the idea of being traumatized can add to the trauma rather than help deal with it. Others suggest the critical need to validate traumatic events. A focus on capacity, resilience, or vitality should not prevent acknowledgment of trauma, but rather harness individuals' or groups' strengths to deal with their experiences.

Trauma-informed care is a growing approach that, far from reinforcing trauma, requires professionals to recognize the impact of traumatic experiences on their clients, just as cultural safety requires sensitivity to and recognition of their unique needs. 'Patients with a history of traumatic life events can become distressed or re-traumatized as the result of healthcare experiences. These patients can benefit from trauma-informed care that is sensitive to their unique needs' (Reeves, 2015, p. 698).

> **Scenario**
> 2021 marked the 76th anniversary of the end of the Holocaust for Jewish people. Olga Horak was one of the last survivors of Auschwitz, the Nazi Concentration camp where the murder of over a million people took place during World War II. Concentration camps forcibly contained those that the Nazi regime targeted on the basis of religion, ethnicity, sexual orientation, disability, or political beliefs. In a television interview, Olga said in response to the idea of 'getting over the past': 'People say, 'Live for the future, don't live in the past'. But I don't live in the past … the past lives in *me*' (The Project, 2 February 2021).
>
> > In the History chapter we looked at how the past influences the present and the future. What other examples can you think of where a client's past *lives in them*?
> >
> > How might this affect someone's health-seeking behaviors?
> >
> > What are some ways that people may respond to different experiences in health care?
>
> What can you do as a health professional to recognize their capacity, resilience, and cultural vitality?

> **Scenario**
> In one particular town, gun violence was recognized as a major issue that health and other authorities wanted to address. A staff member of a human services agency set up a program to tackle gun violence, hoping the community members would engage, but was disappointed when nobody came. She began telling anyone who would listen, 'but *they* need this program!' There had been community meetings beforehand, at which the staff member believed they had an agreement with the community. The staff member concluded in a jaded way, 'they just aren't interested in helping themselves'.
> - What might have influenced the failure of people to engage, even though they agreed it was important?
> - What is it called when someone talks in terms of '*they* don't do this; *they* don't do that'. Where have the professionals positioned themselves relative to the community?
>
> Some weeks later, the staff member met a young mother and asked her why she didn't come to the Gun Violence program when she had been someone who agreed it was important for her community. She responded that she would have liked to attend but had no transport and no one to look after her children because the program was to be held in the evening.
>
> - How could this program have been managed differently?
> - What other strategies could be used to harness the capacity and resilience of the community? Think about multipronged approaches and strategies. Could she engage the mother to talk to others in her area, for example? The professional in this case could be more of a facilitator of engagement rather than have the project rely on them.

Changing the Discourse

Much of the literature related to certain groups presents a bleak picture, and this is justifiable as long as we have disparities. Many groups are frequently and historically referred to in terms of their perceived deficits, disadvantages and what is believed to be lacking. It is our contention that deficits, disadvantages, and lacking therefore inevitably become the 'norm'. When the dominant discourse confirms this view, it becomes almost an unchallenged 'truth' that often goes without critique.

As health and human services professionals, it may therefore be useful to challenge current and past discourses or ways of talking about and framing the issues. If individuals and organizations can begin unpacking their own histories and constructions of certain groups, then it may be possible to develop new and more hopeful discourses. Consider the article, 'The social determinants of being an Indigenous non-smoker' (Thomas et al., 2008). These researchers specifically focus on the variables associated with being a nonsmoker, rather than on being a smoker, to change the emphasis to those of resilience and wellness rather than of deficit and illness. Think back to the chapter on Consuming Research. How much research is usually focused on negatives rather than examining the conditions that support individuals and groups to avoid high-risk health behaviors?

> **Scenario**
> A small rural community had a problem with youth misusing substances. A community nurse tried to engage those youth in having health checks so set up a night of movies, burgers, and milkshakes to encourage their attendance, which worked well for a number of weeks. After a month, however, youth who had not been engaged in misusing substances began to pretend that they were so they too could get free burgers and a movie.
> - What do you think had happened?
> - What unintended message was being given by the health professional to those that did not misuse substances?
> - How could this have been done differently?
>
> Rather than target those who succumbed to substance misuse, there may have been an opportunity to engage those youth who didn't misuse substances to involve them in the program as peer mentors or role models. It is a necessary skill for professionals to examine what might be an unintended message in their approach. For those youth who did not misuse substances, the unintended message was that there was a 'reward' for engaging in harmful activities. You got attention.

There has been a small but increasing call for reorienting the language around health in other parts of the world. Now may be a tipping point in the way U.S. citizens, and health and human services professionals, in particular, construct and choose to talk about individuals and communities. Obviously, we need to do more than simply change the words we use, and we are not suggesting that the solutions are found only in the language we use. But as the issues of identity and labelling have indicated, how we choose to talk about people—any people—reveals much about our underlying thoughts, attitudes, and beliefs. We suggest that unless there is a dominant culture change in the discourses of inherent disadvantage and deficit, health will remain constrained by low expectations and 'truths' that create outcomes contrary to what is desired—that is, equitable health for all Americans.

Forgiveness and Reconciliation

Throughout this book, we have learned about many forms of harm and violence inflicted on people, their families, and communities. These harms can be expressed through us in our behaviors and in the form of various illnesses, whether mental, emotional, or physical. While a great deal of effort goes toward healing in the form of medical and health services or through social or mental health services, less effort has gone into forgiveness and reconciliation work. While this kind of work may formerly have been viewed as withing the domain of religious or spiritual approaches, there is a growing interest and body of scholarly work advocating for reconciliation or forgiveness as ways to heal.

> **Video**
> Watch the following video about one man's way of dealing with his mother's murder at the hands of his father.
> https://www.youtube.com/watch?v=wPddhhNcXHw. Accessed July 7, 2021 and the title is: Son forgives father 32 years after watching him kill his mother.

> What do you think of forgiveness as a form of capacity and resilience? How might reconciliation or forgiveness work become more a part of culturally safe health and human services practice?

> **Making It Local**
> Can you find examples of inspirational people or community groups that demonstrate resilience, capacity, and/or cultural vitality in your state or local area? What are the specific traits or attributes that make them inspirational?
> How might you harness these strengths in your practice with clients who may be facing major health challenges?

Traditional Knowledges

Far too often, Indigenous peoples, Black Americans, and other people in the U.S. are positioned as in need of help and education. From the chapter on History, we discussed how many of the health problems facing people today can be directly linked to the radical change in circumstances brought about by the experiences of colonization. Prior to the arrival of Europeans, Indigenous Peoples and Black Americans, forced from their homelands, had their own medicinal knowledge, doctors, midwives, societal laws for reducing risk of ill-health and injury, and diets that were balanced and energy efficient. This knowledge is still accessible although undoubtedly there has been considerable loss of teachers and holders of some of this knowledge. It is not our place as non-Indigenous authors to present others' intellectual property. There are excellent publications and resources produced by Indigenous communities that we encourage readers to explore. For our purposes, however, look at the following scenario and reflect on your responses to it.

> **Scenario**
> Nancy had a serious diabetic ulcer on her foot that would not heal. Doctors advised her that she would need a partial amputation. Many people in the health care teams talked with her about the need to amputate, but Nancy just smiled at them and said there was no need. The health team initially felt Nancy was in denial about her own health. However, when they spoke further with Nancy, they found out she came from a long line of traditional healers. Nancy had decided to try a traditional medicine, applying a thick paste of a compound made from local plants around her community. Many people, including family members, continued to encourage Nancy to have the operation recommended by the doctors, because they had seen other family members pass away from sepsis from diabetic ulcers. Several years later Nancy still has her foot, and the ulcer has completely healed. She attributes it not only to the traditional medicine itself, but also to her unwavering belief in her own cultural knowledge.
> - What does this scenario say about the strengths and/or limitations of western medicine?
> - Why are traditional medicines not researched and used more widely?
> - How would you have responded to Nancy when she informed you that she wanted to delay surgery to try her own treatment?
>
> We are not suggesting that the outcome would be the same for everyone, although pharmaceutical companies have been trying to access rights and intellectual property from Indigenous peoples globally for a long time. What we are suggesting is that Western medicine does not always hold all the answers and we should be open to other knowledges. Also, the link between mind and body has been well established. Nancy's belief in her medicines is no different or less valid than belief in Western medications and treatments.

Professionals, when being mindful of power differentials with clients, may find better job satisfaction and improved engagement when approaching their practice as partners rather than authorities. For some professionals, there can be a hostile reaction to individuals who may have found information about their health issue in a 'Google search'. Rather than being threatened or affronted by someone having done some pre-reading, a culturally safe approach would involve recognizing the client's capacity to seek out information, including alternative viewpoints. Professionals have an opportunity in such a situation to check the client's understanding, the quality of the information they obtained and to engage in dialogue that doesn't diminish their fears or anxieties. 'Tell me what you've read and let's talk about it...' rather than 'Look, I'm the expert here'.

> **Activity**
> Read the following poem on one person's way of dealing with historical trauma.
> **Poem**
> *Stretch marks*, By Whisper Young
>> So she asked me about my stretch marks and I told her baby girl these are from carrying greatness
>> And when you're compressing coal into diamonds it's more than blatant
>> That the epidermis isn't granted much patience
>> See you? You're to be the cure for hatred
>> Why my body purged mine till shaken
>> As you grew till my ankles became swollen and I felt my back was literally breaking
>> So I stretched till the abdominal aesthetics of an athletic lifetime were depleted
>> So I stretched till my crown was fully polished and my nurturing gardens were fully weeded
>> I stretched until my perfect frame was deleted
>> My selfishness was superseded
>> Wisdom gathered and heeded
>> Young Queen you were the best thing I never knew I needed
>> More precious than the most ancient Egyptian jewel
>> Too serious for scholars to master in the most Ivy League of schools
>> You were my cargo and I needed to carry you like the wisdom of a centennial
>> I was required to carry you like
>> Mothers with bleeding feet carrying their bundles by starlight
>> Refusing to allow chattel slavery to be a part of their children's birthright
>> Like
>> Yeshua carried his cross through the streets to give up his own life
>> For his persecutors despite
>> Child
>> You are the Ancestor's smile
>> Why they held their peace, all the while being reviled
>> The reason for their determination
>> The Most High's presentation
>> Of answers to the prayers and supplication of all of creation

> What many never got to see 'pon this earth but more than hoped for
> Why they knew their return to greatness was more than folklore
> You are royalty and so much more
> And I stretched because EVERYTHING great The Most High ever breathed was packaged in
> Ancestors from many nations in addition to African
> See these are the marks caused by the rebirthing of champions
> When they leave behind the heavenly crossing over to this life these are their footprints
> A reminder of the duties of birthing magnificence
> So I stretched
> And stretched
> And stretched
> And I'll stretch even more to raise it
> Stretch marks....
>
> **Reflection**
>
> - In what ways does the *Stretch Marks* poem illustrate capacity and resilience?
> - How does the author illustrate transgenerational suffering and traumas? How do these traumas become 'embodied'?
> - Through this poem, what is the purpose of the suffering?

PTSD, or Post-Traumatic Stress Disorder, is a psychiatric diagnosis for a range of symptoms that can occur following a traumatic event such as nightmares, frequent thinking about the event, irritability, difficulty concentrating, etc. Researchers identified that many people who experience traumatic events or experiences can also develop a range of positive, or life-enhancing 'symptoms', such as improved relationships, feelings of radical acceptance, an overall transformation in one's sense of purpose, a greater enthusiasm and interest in life and others, and a deeper sense of spirituality or oneness with the world. This is called Post-Traumatic Growth.

How do the concepts of PTSD and Post-Traumatic Growth relate to the deficits-based approaches versus the strengths-based perspective? How do these ideas relate to capacity and resilience?

In a similar vein, mental health researchers and professionals have explored reducing the deficit focus of Western biomedical and psychiatric approaches to mental illness. The Power Threat Meaning Framework was developed as an alternative approach to trauma or 'threats'.

> The Framework… looks at how we make sense of these experiences and how messages from wider society can increase our feelings of shame, self-blame, isolation, fear and guilt.
>
> The approach of the Framework is summarized in four questions that can apply to individuals, families or social groups:
>
> 1. What has happened to you? (How is power operating in your life?)
> 2. How did it affect you? (What kind of threats does this pose?)
> 3. What sense did you make of it? (What is the meaning of these situations and experiences to you?)
> 4. What did you have to do to survive? (What kinds of threat responses are you using?)
>
> Two further questions help us think about what skills and resources people might have and how they might pull all these ideas and responses together into a personal narrative or story:
>
> 1. What are your strengths? (What access to Power resources do you have?)
> 2. What is your story? (How does all this fit together?) (The British Psychological Society, n.d.).

Success Stories

One of the best ways to obtain an idea of capacity and resilience is to look at a few 'success stories'—programs that have been initiated by or have involved the intended participants. In this short video, First Nations people talk about 'How Bison Restoration Seeks to Heal the Quapaw Nation'. https://www.youtube.com/watch?v=E5fQBV0FWCM.

This video starts with the premise: 'Their resilience is our resilience' and goes on to describe the symbiotic relationship with the buffalo as necessary to restore the health of land, and people. It also debunks the myth of people 'losing' their culture. 'Our tribes aren't dying. We're contemporary, we're here…' There is pride in continuing cultural vitality and sharing knowledge.

In watching the video in full, you will also see further examples of the dispossession and decimation of the Quapaw peoples who were forcibly removed from what is now Arkansas and relocated to land that was thought to be worthless but later found to be rich in ore. However, the colonization of the Quapaw was far from over, when the U.S. Bureau of Indian Affairs tried to bypass legalities and allowed external interests to profit from the ore, leaving decades of toxic waste. In 1993, 34% of children had lead levels above Federal limits. The Quapaw are the only tribe now to receive funding from the Environmental Protection Agency (EPA) to clean up. Now under a policy of self-determination and self-government, the Quapaw have determined that the buffalo are necessary to help remediate land, acknowledging that they are 'all we have left, all we have been able to hang onto'.

- How would you respond to someone who told you that their well-being was tied to the existence of bison?
- What principles of cultural safety are evident in this approach to health promotion?

Cultural sensitivity, a precursor to cultural safety suggests that we may not hold the same beliefs as those we engage with, but that we need to respect the right to hold differing beliefs. Often it is not as different as might be imagined. What role does the buffalo play environmentally? How do they differ from domestic cattle?

Think about your own health beliefs? Revisit your own definition of health. What do you practice that is reflective of your own culture that may be health-promoting or enhancing?

Websites

Below are two websites that illustrate strength-based approaches for building community capacity and resilience:

Forward Promise. This is an approach to promoting the health of boys and young men of color. https://forwardpromise.org/.

Qungasvik Toolbox: A toolbox for promoting youth sobriety and reasons for living in Yup'ik/Cup'ik communities. https://www.sprc.org/

> resources-programs/qungasvik-toolbox-toolbox-promoting-youth-sob riety-reasons-smyliving-yup%E2%80%99ik-cup%E2%80%99ik.
> http://www.qungasvik.org/preview/.
> Note here the language choice in the title of this resource. Rather than calling this a suicide prevention resource, they use a more positive description by 'promoting youth sobriety' and 'reasons for living'.

Black Lives Matter

Before looking at the Black Lives Matter website, jot down some ideas, perhaps even experiences, you have about the Black Lives Matter organization and movement. Write down what you think you know about the movement, the organization, who started it, what it stands for, etc. Now, look at the Black Lives Matter website: https://blacklivesmatter.com/about/. How did your notes before looking at the website, compare with what you learned?

There has been considerable controversy about the organization and the intent behind the Black Lives Matter organization. Read the information on the website. What does it mean to say Black Lives Matter? There are some who have taken this to mean that Black lives matter *more* than other people's lives. It's perhaps easier for some to play word games than to acknowledge what is actually a plea for people to care about a group that has historically been dehumanized and killed without consequence. Saying Black Lives Matter, means they matter *too*, that they should matter as much as any other life. Talking about maternal deaths in Black populations does not mean no other maternal deaths matter or discussing Veteran health does not negate the need for other groups to have their health care needs recognized. Why then might there be such an extreme response to this maxim? Critique the information provided on the website and consider how the idea of Black Lives Matter relates to cultural safety.

> **Making It Local**
> - What are local people in your area doing for the health and well-being for themselves and their community?
> - What key elements can you identify that might contribute to these successes?

Conclusion

Harnessing strengths rather than focusing on perceived deficits is more likely to achieve the goals of empowerment and self-reliance required of a cultural safety approach. There are many positive examples that could be shared nationally. The projects described in this chapter illustrate some of the outcomes that are possible when the discourse is reoriented away from deficits to a focus on strengths and capacity.

References

Dvorsky, M. R., Breaux, R., & Becker, S. P. (2020). Finding ordinary magic in extraordinary times: Child and adolescent resilience during the COVID-19 pandemic. *European Child and Adolescent Psychiatry*. https://doi.org/10.1007/s00787-020-01583-8.

Eckermann, A., Dowd, T., Nixon, L., Chong, E., Gray, R., & Johnson, S. (2010). *Binah Goonj: Bridging cultures in Aboriginal health*. Churchill Livingstone Elsevier.

Lalonde, C. E. (2006). Identity formation and cultural resilience in aboriginal communities. In R. J. Flynn, P. Dudding, & J. Barber (Eds.), *Promoting resilience in child welfare* (pp. 52–71). University of Ottawa Press.

Luthar, S. (2003). *Resilience and vulnerability: Adaptation in the context of childhood adversities*. Cambridge University Press.

Masten, A. S. (2001). Ordinary magic: Resilience processes in development. *American Psychologist, 56*(3), 227–238. https://doi.org/10.1037/0003-066X.56.3.227.

Reeves, E. (2015). A synthesis of the literature on trauma-informed care. *Issues in Mental Health Nursing, 36*(9), 698–709. https://doi.org/10.3109/016 12840.2015.1025319.

The British Psychological Society. (n.d.). *Introduction to the PTFM*. https:// www.bps.org.uk/power-threat-meaning-framework/introduction-ptmf.

Thomas, D. P., Briggs, V., Anderson, I. P. S., & Cunningham, J. (2008). Social determinants of being an Indigenous non-smoker. *Australian and New Zealand Journal of Public Health, 32*(2), 110–116.

Wallerstein, N. (1992). Powerlessness, empowerment and health: Implications for health promotion programs. *American Journal of Health Promotion, 6*, 197–205.

11

Intercultural Communication

In this chapter, *Intercultural Communication,* we explore a variety of case studies related to healthcare communications. Conflicting worldviews and miscommunication are major challenges when professionals differ in cultural and linguistic background from the clients in their care. This chapter provides an opportunity to examine intercultural interactions in various practice settings, as well as exploring what it means to 'decolonize' practice. Health literacy as both an individual and organizational responsibility is discussed as an important element of cultural safety.

Chapter Objectives

After completing this chapter, you should be able to:

- demonstrate awareness of own language use
- describe some intercultural interactions that may influence practice and healthcare outcomes

- identify factors that facilitate or hinder communication between health professionals and patients who differ in cultural and linguistic backgrounds
- develop strategies to decolonize intercultural interactions
- define health literacy and identify strategies for enhancing health literacy in practice.

Intercultural or Cross-Cultural Interactions

As stated from the outset, all cultures and peoples are diverse and have diversity within. If we were all the same there would be no need to examine our interactions at all. However, in the healthcare and human services settings, the potential to misread, misinterpret, or miscommunicate leaves both practitioners and clients vulnerable to unintended negative consequences.

Cultural safety starts with *awareness* of difference. In doing so, we hopefully become aware of the commonalities between groups as well. For some, recognizing differences in the first place may be inhibited by being culturally blinkered—an inability to see beyond one's own cultural norms. This can get in the way of knowledge development and understandings needed to move to sensitivity and safety.

In this chapter, we provide examples of effective, and not so effective, ways of interacting. We strongly caution readers to recognize that not all communication can or should fit a neat stereotype. However, developing some language awareness can be a useful step in developing culturally safe communications.

Communication in Health and Human Services

An essential starting point for looking at any intercultural communication is to examine your own communication. Do you know how you communicate? What are your normal modes of asking questions, showing attention, or clarifying? What is polite and impolite in your own primary language? If you are uncertain, think about it. If, for example, your primary language is English, start to pay attention to how English operates. English is spoken widely throughout the world and yet varies significantly across cultural groups. Encounters in health care or human services are often stressful for clients and when this is further aggravated by a language or communication difference between provider and client, the outcomes can range from frustrating to fatal.

In their now classic study, researchers Beckman and Frankel (1984) found when looking at communication in doctors' visits, only 23% of patients were able to finish their explanations and it only took 18 seconds, on average, for the doctor to interrupt. That is when a common language is spoken, so what happens when there is a language difference? It's not surprising when you look at the culture of the healthcare environment. It's often time-poor, resource-poor, and pressured but there is also an explanation that stems from how English is used.

English as a language does not handle silences well. It's a language that can be rapid and silence within spoken communication invites a response, but when someone is a speaker of another language, silences may mean something else. Silence created from the time needed for translating between languages, silence as a way of showing thoughtfulness about a question, or even silence as a way to show reluctance to answer a question are all ways to communicate something. The professional cultures of health and human services, however, is such that time is considered something we don't have enough of—'I haven't got time to wait'—yet getting communication wrong with patients could mean that more time is spent later with poor outcomes.

Frankel and Stein (1999) describe four habits—invest in the beginning, elicit the client's perspective, demonstrate empathy, and invest in the end—based on research evidence for improved outcomes in care. Although these have been designed for the medical or general practitioner, they may be useful for any health or human services professional to employ when working with any client. Commonly, there is the need for a polite introduction—checking that the participants are all safe in terms of the convenience of the interaction.

Invest in the beginning—listen to the reason the client is there. It is important to allow time for greetings and rapport building before getting straight to the business. To believe that we do not have time for these simple processes is a false economy. What is saved by being so time efficient that you end up with wrong or poorer quality information exchange?

Let the client finish. Elicit the client's perspective—this is about asking the client what *they* think the problem is or what *they* think the solution might be. Clients have often thought about the problem before coming to see a professional and have already developed ideas about what the problem is and what might be the solution. This does not mean you have nothing to offer. They have after all, come to you for your expertise and assistance. It simply means you can also find out what the client's concerns are and deal with those concerns—such as fears of cancer or concerns about the adverse effects of medication. It allows for a richer picture to emerge. It is also an opportunity to validate the client's own worldview and belief system and offer service that is not at the expense of these aspects. Everyone is the expert of their own lives and their own experiences. Clients may well have talked to others and maybe even done some of their own research on their symptoms and experiences before coming to see you. The investment that they have made to understand what they are going through is valuable information that will help you provide more accurate as well as culturally safe service.

Empathy is about showing compassion. We can reflect on various 'clues' from the client to indicate how they are feeling. Sometimes, unfortunately, empathy can be more easily provided to those of a similar cultural background to the practitioner. Those of a different cultural background may receive less empathy without the practitioner being conscious of possible differing responses. This is another important reason to engage in critical reflective practice.

The Influence of Accents on Communications

Who reading this book does not have an accent? So, think about what the following statement implies: *'I had trouble understanding him because he spoke with an accent'*.

- Reflect on the above statement. What assumptions have been made?
- Who is positioned as 'normal' and who is 'different'?
- Who has the perceived deficit?

There are some significant differences across the U.S. in terms of accents or dialects, even among those who speak only English. In some regions, accents or dialects are so distinct as to potentially lead to misunderstandings. English-speaking professionals' lack of familiarity with specific pronunciations can lead to great frustration, on both sides, as well as shame and avoidance of certain situations. The consequences of these can range from an amusing encounter to something far more serious.

Remember the discussions around identity and the importance of our names. For many speakers of languages other than English, it's not uncommon that names are changed by health, or education professionals who might be unfamiliar and unskilled in pronouncing certain names: 'Oh, that's a hard one, I think I'll just call you Betty– is that OK with you?' Have you or anyone you know had to change your name or had it changed by someone who could not pronounce it properly?

- What message does this give the client about how you perceive them?
- How is this potentially a colonizing act?
- What would be the culturally safe approach to your difficulty with pronouncing someone's name?

The issue of frustration and embarrassment in trying to make oneself understood is a major issue for some people. In the U.S. today, there is an expectation that most people will or should speak English and therefore have no real problem with communication in a healthcare setting. However, this is a serious underestimation of what many authors believe to be a major barrier to safe and effective health care (Osborne, 2018).

The lack of awareness of potential communication barriers can often result in clients being labelled 'non-compliant', 'non-communicative', 'non-responsive', or not interested in their own health. This labeling locates responsibility for outcomes on the clients. It is rarely acknowledged that the healthcare services need to examine their own responsibility for communication failures. How likely is it, for example, for a note in a client file to read something like this?

'*Note: Ineffective client history obtained due to poor cross-cultural communication skills of staff. Further staff education required.*'

Website and Reading

Explore the PBS website, '*Do you speak American?*' https://www.pbs.org/speak/ for information on dialects and language in the U.S. See the section *American Varieties* under the section *From Sea to Shining Sea* where you will find information on African American English, Cajun, Chicano English, Pittsburghese, and more. https://www.pbs.org/speak/seatosea/americanvarieties/.

You might also like to read this article for more about dialects in the U.S. and to explore a map of dialects across the country: Wilson, R. (2013, December 2). What dialect do you speak? A map of American English. *The Washington Post*. https://www.washingtonpost.com/blogs/govbeat/wp/2013/12/02/what-dialect-to-do-you-speak-a-map-of-american-english/.

The Fluency Corp provides some useful communication tips on their website relating to American English dialects: https://fluencycorp.com/american-english-dialects/.

Think about the requirements of 'informed consent' for many medical procedures. When working with patients whose first language is not English, if put to the test of what constitutes informed consent, there would be many examples that would fail the standard. How can you be certain that a client has truly understood what they are consenting to, what the procedures are, and what the risks are? Even when someone's first language is English, this is often difficult to determine. The social elements of obtaining consent, often in rushed circumstances, are less than ideal.

Communication challenges with linguistically diverse clients have also been identified as a major stressor for staff, who often feel unprepared and experience a sense of 'hopelessness'. Of greatest concern is the idea that preventable morbidity and mortality result from something that should be more easily facilitated these days. So why has communication been so neglected as an issue of consequence?

What can be done in practice? Without creating a tick-box approach, there are aspects of communication patterns worth examining in relation to English structures and patterns. More precisely, there are elements of English language that professionals can be made aware of in order to recognize where potential communication barriers might occur. Cultural safety starts with an awareness of one's own culture and the potential differences between the practitioner and the consumer. Below in Table 11.1 is a brief introduction to 'language awareness' that focuses on key elements of communication.

While it would be nice if everyone followed such prescribed ways of interacting, the variables that individuals bring to an encounter are extensive, which is why such a checklist is offered with caution. These are just a few aspects that you might encounter, where English could be creating expectations of understanding that are not there.

Limited English Proficiency (LEP)

Dettenmeier (2014) defines a person with Limited English Proficiency (LEP) as an 'individual whose primary language isn't English and who has a limited ability to read, write, speak, and understand English'. While this sounds like a deficit, it should be remembered that speaking your first language is not a limitation and effective communication in healthcare and human services is a human right. Surveys indicate that about 80% of people in the U.S. speak only English at home. However, 20% speak mainly languages other than English and many speak multiple languages. Of the 20% of those who speak a language other than English at home, a significant proportion don't speak English well and some not at all. These ratios are expected to increase in the future with changes to patterns of migration.

Table 11.1 Elements of healthcare communications in the U.S

Question formats	To indicate a question in English, there is often a raised intonation at the end. 'Do you have any children?' (the voice tone rises on children.) Not all languages do this and may sound like a statement when conversing in English as a second or other language 'I need to bring my children?' can in fact be a question without the obvious rise
Use of medical jargon	Use of technical language or jargon is often considered professional and used for specificity within practice. It indicates knowledge and expertise. However, when used in communications with patients, it becomes a barrier for conversing with lay people and particularly LEP clients. Use of jargon without awareness or regard can also be used to enhance the power of the users and exclude others. A decolonizing approach is one which limits or makes sure to explain medical terminology so the client is well-informed This can be done by linking technical words to commonly used words or terms E.g.: So, do you have any problems with *diabetes*, sugar sickness? Have you ever been tested for sugar or what we sometimes call *glucose* in your blood?

Model appropriate English	There is a distinction between plain English and over-simplifying that also needs to consider the age and responsibility of the client

Substandard English doesn't help understanding yet this is something English speakers often do when they are talking with someone of a different language background. You may need to slow down a little, and use plain language, but your English should remain standard |
| The use of silence | In the U.S, when using English, questions bring an expectation of a prompt answer. For some other language speakers, questions, even seemingly routine ones, require careful consideration as a matter of good manners, which is demonstrated by lengthy pauses. Such pauses can be disconcerting to people whose first language is English. They may interpret silence as a failure to understand or as resistance to answering, or even dishonesty. Apart from a politeness, pauses may also reflect the time taken to process information into the person's first language and then relay the answer back in English. Try not to interrupt and allow adequate time for responses |

(continued)

Table 11.1 (continued)

The use of abstract concepts	Healthcare often involves the use of abstract concepts that are difficult to translate, for example 'anxiety', 'depression', or even 'pain'. Ask instead what the point of the concept is and what needs to be done about it. For example, instead of asking someone how much pain they are in, ask them, 'What would you like for your pain?' English also uses metaphors or similes to explain abstract concepts which can be confusing for speakers of a different language. You can't assume that an example you use with an English speaker will be interpreted in the same way for speakers of other languages
Body language	English speakers use body language less consciously than some other language speakers, who incorporate gestures and facial expressions into the communication. Interpretation of facial gestures and non-verbal responses can be culturally specific Many cultures use non-verbal communication to convey information. When asking a question, health staff may 'miss' the non-verbal answer that was given by the client. Eye contact is also a feature of English communications in the U.S. that shows interest and honesty, whereas some cultures avoid eye contact at times, to show respect depending on who is speaking and what the topic is about

Reluctance to make a decision or 'yes' response	In English, to say yes to something implies and agreement. Some cultural communication styles use concurrence: that is, to agree with the person, and then continue on with no expectation of agreement. It can be impolite to contradict or confront, so agreement does not necessarily oblige one to do something, even if they have said they would For example, you might have asked someone to wait for something and they reply yes, but then you notice later, they have left. This can be frustrating in a healthcare setting. A helpful strategy might be to ask a little more, about how waiting might impact: "Do you need to be somewhere else, -is someone able to watch your children while you're here?' This might help gain more confidence about the response or indicate an issue requiring further attention

When professionals are not provided with the skills and resources for working with clients who have Limited English Proficiency, this puts both clients and professionals at risk of miscommunications, especially when healthcare and human services environments are almost exclusively limited to only English. A background of language difference between provider and client can result in shorter consultations, less access to preventative health services, poor medication and treatment compliance, medical errors, and more. Remember that with a cultural safety approach, the onus for communication is on the providers and the systems in which they work.

While many health and human services have tried implementing services for people for whom their primary language is not English, these are not consistently available in all areas. Dettenmeier (2014) advises that there are certain documents that must be translated according to Health and Human Services guidelines. These documents are vital to patients' healthcare and include: consent and complaint forms, documents that must be provided by law, notices about emergency preparedness and risk communications notices of eligibility for benefits, and notices about no-cost language assistance.

Providing culturally safe care requires services and professionals to find resources and strategies to help them communicate most effectively with clients, and it is important that these resources be critiqued to ensure their safety as well as effectiveness. It's a positive thing to learn some phrases for simple instructions in a different language, but it is also limited, and may still lead to misunderstanding and error. Using graphics or pictures is similarly limited and needs to be checked for their interpretation, but of course, these can be helpful communication aids. What is not helpful is speaking a substandard form of English, or childlike English (as opposed to plain, simple English) or raising the volume of your voice when speaking with clients.

Let us preface this by saying once again that people's life experiences need to be thoughtfully considered and we need to be careful not to act on stereotyped notions. The use of broken or substandard English by English-speaking professionals does not enhance understanding and can be demeaning. But there may be times when simplifying English is necessary to facilitate understanding. Be mindful of the experience of the recipient of care. If you are not sure if your communication is understood, ask the client or family or support people with them to repeat what it is they have understood. In addition, it may help to explain why you are asking with something like, 'Could you tell me what I just said so I can be sure that I've explained everything properly?' This brief rationale shifts the responsibility to the practitioner who needs to make sure that their communication is effective, rather than placing the responsibility on the client.

With anyone of a linguistically different background, you cannot simply check understanding by asking yes/no questions. A plain English approach (not simple or childlike English) will facilitate greater understanding between yourself and clients of most backgrounds. Similarly, the use of technical jargon may be another barrier to understanding for many clients.

> **Scenario**
> 'A nine-year old Vietnamese girl died from a reaction to the drug Reglan. Her parents primarily spoke Vietnamese, yet no competent interpreter was used throughout the child's encounters with the medical system. Instead, records show the patient and her 16-year-old brother served as interpreters. In the subsequent lawsuit, an expert witness who was a professional interpreter testified that "the parents were not able to adequately understand and address [the patient's] medical needs—the failure of the doctor and the facility to provide a professional medical interpreter was a substantial factor in causing [patient]'s death"' (Health IT Outcomes, 2014).
> - What are the laws around providing access to interpreters for LEP patients?
> - What are the key elements of informed consent?
> - Discuss the ethical issues in using family as interpreters?
> - What strategies are helpful when using an interpreter?
> - What cultural safety principles should be applied in scenarios like this?

Think of a situation where you have had difficulty communicating. Perhaps you travelled to a country where the primary language was not your first language. Maybe you can recall a situation of trying to understand a different professional area and not understanding what they were talking about—perhaps trying to understand an economist or geologist, when economics or geology was not your area of knowledge or familiarity.

- What was your experience? What communication skills did you rely on? These may have included nonverbal cues which themselves may not be universally understood.

Think about an experience of needing to communicate with a client whose first language was not English.

- How effective was your communication?
- What do you expect of clients when they come for a healthcare encounter?
- What do you expect of clients who may not speak English as their first language?
- What do you do or use to assist communications?
- How aware are you of the issues affecting communication for some Americans?

> **Scenario**
> 'A first responder in Florida misinterpreted a single Spanish word, *intoxicado*, to mean "intoxicated" rather than its intended meaning of "feeling sick to the stomach, or nauseated." This led to a delay in diagnosis, which resulted in a potentially preventable case of quadriplegia, and ultimately, a $71 million malpractice settlement' (Graves, 2015).
> **Critical Thinking**
> - Without knowing all the aspects of the above case, reflect on how such a situation may have arisen.
> - What actions might have changed such an outcome?
> - What policies and procedures might be developed to ensure such a tragedy never occurs again?

Working with Interpreters

It is surprising how often professionals will fail to engage an interpreter when these services are available, especially in an area as critical as healthcare communications. Sometimes clients themselves will resist involving interpreters for a range of reasons. But sometimes, professionals believe that they either don't have the time or that they communicate 'well enough' or the client understands 'well enough'. What do you think of this standard for healthcare communications? Medical interpreting specifically is a specialized skill and when health professionals upskill themselves to work effectively with interpreters, this can only lead to better outcomes for clients. What is the role of health professionals for whom their primary language is not English? There may be many health and human services professionals who can speak languages other than English, but they are not necessarily trained for medical interpreting work and to do so may compromise the cultural safety of an encounter. What responsibility does healthcare and human services have for preparing all staff for culturally safe communication?

Confidentiality is another concern within health and human service communications. However, in respect of culturally preferred ways of operating, it may be that the client wishes to have family or other support people with them who are entitled and expected to be involved in information exchanges. The important thing is not to assume these entitlements exist and to check with the client about who they wish to include in communications.

Singleton and Krause (2009) offer some insights into intercultural healthcare communications:

> Even when an interpreter is used to facilitate understanding, or when a patient for whom English is a second language appears to have competent speaking and listening skills in English, cultural issues may still interfere with the effectiveness of communication between the patient and a healthcare provider. For example, many cultures emphasize showing politeness and deference toward healthcare providers who are perceived as authority figures. High context cultures have a preference for indirect, non-confrontational styles of communication; a cultural preference for

conflict avoidance can lead patients to say what they believe the healthcare provider wants them to say, or voice agreement or understanding whether or not they actually agree or understand. Asking questions and self-advocating in high context cultures might not be acceptable. Sometimes culture even influences which healthcare provider(s) a patient or family member will listen to and/or speak with. For example, there may be a preference for listening to a doctor over a nurse, or a male over a female. These cultural preferences can influence a patient's listening and speaking practices in clinical encounters. (Singleton & Krause, 2009)

> **Activity**
> Look up high context and low context cultures. Where do you position yourself in terms of these descriptions?
> Check your local area or your workplace for interpreter services. How easy are these to find? Have you worked with interpreters? What culturally safe considerations might be useful in working with an interpreter?

Health Literacy

Health literacy has received less attention than it perhaps should as it contributes to health inequalities. Some 60% of all Americans, regardless of their primary language, experience poor health literacy at times, affecting medication adherence, compliance with medical instructions, and treatment outcomes. Not only is there potential for misunderstandings due to cross-cultural communication, but the way individuals and groups conceptualize and use health information influences the exchange of health information. Research suggests that there is a strong link between health and literacy, with literacy skills able to predict health status more strongly than age, income, employment status, educational level, and racial or ethnic group. Although literacy is implicit, health literacy is more than simply the ability to read and write. Low health literacy is more likely (but not exclusively) to occur in those with low general literacy, the elderly, those with impaired eyesight, hearing, and mental alertness, some ethnic and cultural groups, as well as those on a low-income level.

Low health literacy affects the ability to follow instructions, provide informed consent, take medications, understand disease-related information, learn about disease prevention and self-management, and understand their rights. It affects access and uptake of care and increases the chances of dying of chronic and communicable diseases as well as the costs of health care. As health literacy is about a conceptual understanding, it is important that as practitioners you make sure you are using the same 'language', that is, that you have the same picture in your head as the client. This applies even when people share the same cultural background. Where there is a cultural difference, it is even more critical that you ensure a common understanding before proceeding with any other information exchange.

For example, to ask a client how many cups of coffee, wine, beer, soft drink they might have in a day requires an understanding of how that drink is consumed. For the authors, a cup of coffee may be something around 250 ml or 8 oz. For others, depending on their circumstances, the 'cup' may be a 'grande' holding about 500 mls or 16 oz. So, is it a cup of coffee… or a *cup* of coffee? Are you a 'social drinker or a *social* drinker'? What can help the exchange, if there is any uncertainty, is to have actual examples handy of each sized drinking cup. Here are some suggestions for improving the health literacy of your clients:

- Review written materials—check readability. Most word processing programs have a readability tool under the grammar and spelling check. Look at the reading age and ask yourself if the resource could be stated more plainly. Writing something in a plain way will be more accessible to a wider audience than something written at a college level.
- Use age-appropriate resources—try not to offer adults information that is normally targeted at children, such as pediatric pain tools, unless these have been validated for specific groups.
- Use or develop culturally appropriate, 'local' resources where possible. Without reinventing the wheel, it is helpful to show a resource from

elsewhere to key advisors and then work with them to develop a local resource that will help with engagement and interpretation.
- Lift the standard of expectation—plain English does not have to be simple or childlike English.
- Find a relatable concept from within patients' worldview or experience.
- Use the professional language in tandem with plain/local terms. Talking about diabetes, for example, it is helpful to link the common or lay terminology from the local context, to say something like: 'So tell me about your sugar problems, your *diabetes* …'
- Use graphics, symbols, drawings, illustrations rather than cartoons depending upon the intended audience. Photo-shopped images are a good way of using real pictures and transforming them into graphics. (Check symbols for interpretation because graphics that may represent a tree in some regions may look nothing like a tree in the clients' cultural context.)
- Never assume strong health literacy based on general literacy or educational level.
- Look for signs of low English literacy, such as clients who may avoid reading information in front of you, saying things like they have 'left their glasses at home' and will take the form home to do later.
- Ensure an environment of trust and safety.
- Communicate without jargon.
- Give clients a chance to tell their story without interruption.
- Limit the number of new concepts introduced (three per visit). (Adapted from Harvard T.H. Chan School of Public Health, 2019).

Low health literacy, cultural barriers, and limited English proficiency have been coined the 'triple threat' to effective health communication by The Joint Commission (Schyve, 2007). Health literacy, both conceptually and in practice, has often been siloed from interventions designed to overcome cultural and linguistic barriers (Singleton & Krause, 2009).

Health literacy is not dependent upon written literacy, even though there can be an association. A person who has limited English literacy may have strong health literacy, just as a person with strong English literacy can possess limited health literacy. For example, talking to clients about restricting their fluid intake relies on a shared picture of what fluid is exactly. A client may tell you that they have not had more fluid, just some orange juice. In the intercultural domain, this potential for mismatched ideas is greater. A key principle of cultural safety is to talk with and to the client. Developing health literacy can only enhance the intercultural information exchange.

> **Website**
> An excellent resource for learning more about health literacy can be found at: www.healthliteracy.com.
>
> Health literacy expert, Helen Osborne, publishes a monthly newsletter with tips and strategies for enhancing health literacy both at an individual level and organizationally. She also authored a text, Health Literacy A to Z (2018). Helen has kindly offered readers of this book access to her podcasts, websites, newsletters, including the option to rent or buy digital copies of her textbook. https://redshelf.com/book/1152309/health-literacy-from-a-to-z-2nd-edition-updated-2018-1152309-9781947937130-helen-osborne-medotrl.
>
> Helen's materials often include information for intercultural health literacy as well as for those who speak English as their primary language.

> **Activity**
> Health information given to patients today usually aims to provide plain English explanations. However, the average health information sheet or brochure is presented at a Year 12 reading age. Examine the text below. Even with a readability score of Grade 6, which words and phrases might be difficult for speakers of other languages to read and interpret? Can this be made even plainer without 'dumbing down' the information?
>
> > Asthma has been on the rise all over the world. We need to take action to help people control their asthma. We also need to learn how to prevent asthma. Asthma is a disease of the lungs that cannot be cured. Diseases like asthma that are with us for a long time are called chronic diseases. Asthma, like many chronic diseases, cannot be cured but can be controlled. To understand asthma,

we first have to know some things about our breathing. The airways that move air through our lungs look like an upside down tree. When we breathe in, air flows into our nose and mouth, down our windpipe (trachea), through the air tubes (bronchi) and smaller airways, and into the air sacs (alveoli).

When people have asthma, the airways swell. This swelling causes the airways to become narrow. Also, when people have asthma, mucus builds up in the airways. This swelling (chronic inflammation) and the mucus build-up that goes along with it get in the way of breathing. Medicines can make a difference. (Rudd, et al, 2004).

Try writing your own information sheet. Most word processing programs allow you to check readability levels of written materials by selecting this tool within spelling and grammar check options. Test a few patient information sheets for their readability and, if they are above a 10th-grade level, think about how the information could be made more accessible to readers with a range of reading levels.

How will you know this is appropriate?

Who would you involve in developing the materials?

What elements of culturally safe practice are important to remember when working with clients with different languages and literacy backgrounds than yourself?

Making It Local

Look at the latest policies related to language access in healthcare or human services in your state and nationally. What are the current priorities for health and well-being and how have these been determined? To do this: Go to the following federal government website www.health.gov. Next, go to the relevant state health department site. Search for and download the latest health policy directions or strategies.

Search for any information about language or communication in healthcare and if there is any information about a Patient Bill of Rights. What information can you find?

- Reflect on how these directions fit with the key issues you have been reading about so far in the topic.
- Reflect on what you have noticed either in your own experience in health services or in the context of clinical placements.

- Can you find such a document for your own community?

Conclusion

The content covered in this chapter is offered only as a prompt for what might influence interactions in healthcare settings. It should not be taken as applying to every encounter. The important thing in a cultural safety approach is to find out from the client or from other appropriate resources what the client's unique and specific needs might be. Cultural safety does not offer a checklist of responses. While the aspects discussed in this chapter point to some areas in which culture impacts on interactions; it is important not to see these as prescriptive. Awareness of differences is only a first step along the cultural safety continuum. Acknowledging the right to difference is therefore key to culturally safe communications.

References

Beckman, H. B., & Frankel, R. M. (1984). The effect of physician behavior on the collection of data. *Annals of Internal Medicine, 101,* 692–696.

Dettenmeier, P. A. (2014). ¡Ayúdame! Mi esposo esta inconsciente! No hablo ingles!: Help me! My husband is unconscious! I don't speak English! *Nursing, 44*(6), 60–63. https://doi.org/10.1097/01.NURSE.0000441883.72501.6d PMID: 24841611.

Frankel, R., & Stein, T. (1999). Getting the most out of the clinical encounter: The four habits model. *The Permanente Journal, 3,* 79–88.

Graves, D. (2015). A primer on communication and language assistance. U. S. Department of Health and Human Services, Think Cultural Health. https://thinkculturalhealth.hhs.gov/resources/presentations///a-primer-on-communication-and-language-assistance.

Harvard T. H. Chan School of Public Health. (2019). *Health Literacy Studies Web Site.* www.hsph.harvard.edu/healthliteracy.

Health IT Outcomes. (2014). Nine year old girl dies due to language barrier, interpreting absence at hospital—Stratus video says lack of industry standardization creating healthcare hazard. https://www.healthitoutcomes.com/doc/nine-year-girl-dies-language-hospital-video-healthcare-hazard-0001.

Multicultural Health Communication Service. (n.d.). *Diabetes Fact Sheets.* www.mhcs.health.nsw.gov.au/publicationsandresources/pdf/publication-pdfs/diabetes/5955/doh-5955-eng.pdf.

Osborne, H. (2018). *Health literacy from A to Z: Practical ways to communicate your health message.* Jones and Bartlett.

Rudd, R. E., Zobel, E. K., Fanta, C. H., Surkan, P., Rodriguez-Louis, J., Valderrama, Y., & Daltroy, L. H. (2004). Asthma: In Plain Language. *Health Promotion Practice, 5*(3), 334–340. https://doi.org/10.1177/1524839903257771.

Schyve, P. M. (2007). Language Differences as a Barrier to Quality and Safety in Health Care: The Joint Commission Perspective. *Journal of General Internal Medicine, 22*(2), 360–361.

Singleton, K., & Krause, E. (2009, September 30). Understanding cultural and linguistic barriers to health literacy, *OJIN: The Online Journal of Issues in Nursing.* 14(3), Manuscript 4.

12

Comparable Contexts

In this chapter, *Comparable Contexts,* we will look briefly at the experiences of colonization and race relations in Canada, New Zealand and Australia as well as the U.S.

Colonization impacted Indigenous populations all around the world, both in its impact through 'settlements' and through the enslavement, forced removal and other efforts that led to the forced relocation of people. While there are many similarities in the effects of colonization in various countries, there are also some important differences that can help us to understand what contributes to these impacts and how to move forward. In this chapter, we look more closely at the experiences of colonization and the impacts on health in other comparable nations. This will provide a barometer for evaluating our progress in promoting health equity for Indigenous Peoples and other groups harmed through colonization and colonialism.

Chapter Objectives

After completing this chapter, you should be able to:

- briefly describe the colonizing histories of Australia, Canada, the U.S., and Aotearoa/New Zealand
- understand the health status of colonized peoples in a comparable global context
- explore and critique the transferability of approaches to improving health from other countries with similar histories of colonization
- discuss what is meant by 'engage in a process of decolonization' as health professionals.

Indigenous Peoples in a Comparable Global Context

'There are an estimated 370 million indigenous peoples living in more than 70 countries worldwide. They represent a rich diversity of cultures, religions, traditions, languages and histories; yet continue to be among the world's most marginalized population groups. The health status of indigenous peoples varies significantly from that of non-indigenous population groups in countries all over the world' (WHO, 2007).

We briefly discussed colonialism as it related to the U.S. in the chapter on History. Colonization was certainly not a unique aspect of U.S. history, nor has colonization been limited to British efforts. Many Indigenous Peoples initially welcomed visitors and traders, as had been customary, but when it became clear that these 'visitors' were not in fact intending to leave, colonization took on its destructive form.

If we think of 'colonization' as the process of setting up a colony by a non-Indigenous population, then we can see colonization at a global scale essentially since the beginning of humankind. Colonization is often thought of in terms of colonizing the land, but it includes the impacts on people, such as displacement, enslavement, and genocide. Britain, France, Portugal, Spain, the Netherlands, Belgium, the U.S., and more have colonized other's countries and their peoples in Africa, Asia, the

South Pacific, North, Central and South America, and Europe. Russia and China also have histories of colonization. In fact, few areas on the globe have been unaffected by efforts to colonize people and lands by people from elsewhere.

Historically, colonization has been about gaining resources or finding a new place to live, which has meant dispossessing people of their land, essentially through exerting power over them. Most western accounts rely on singular events signaling the 'beginning' of 'new nations' such as Christopher Columbus 'discovering' America in 1492 and James Cook's 'discovery' of Australia in 1770. However, in most countries, the colonization process was not necessarily a sudden influx of hundreds or thousands of new people suddenly 'moving in'. Rather, it was a gradual process interrelated with other elements, such as contact with 'others' through trade, fishing, and whaling. This gradual process is what sometimes makes understanding the impact of colonization difficult, for both the people who were colonized and those who did the colonizing. It is also important to consider that colonization has not always been a violent process, though violence has characterized much of the colonization that has affected Indigenous Peoples. In fact, one might believe that nonviolent colonizing could be more insidious.

Colonization continues today in forms that may not 'look' like what colonization looked like in the past. Today we see marginalization of various groups, the unequal distribution of wealth and resources, systemic biases in education, law, and health, and a lack of action on climate change that contributes to forced migration. The reality is that few populations have been untouched by colonizing influences, but who benefits and is damaged is important to recognize.

> **Activity**
> - Where are you 'from'? Where did you grow up? Where did your parents grow up? Do you know any history of your family? Where do they 'come from'? Think about where you are today, specifically, where you live, and how you got there, considering your family's history.

> Why did your family move to where they are? Why did your ancestors live where they lived?
> - What is home? How do you understand home and what it means to be 'home'?
> - If your family has lived in the U.S. for at least a few generations, how might the U.S. have changed even since your own parents were children?

Colonization in Australia, the U.S., Canada, and Aotearoa/New Zealand

To examine the effects of colonization, we can look at who the colonizers were, why they were seeking to colonize a new place—what their circumstances were—when the colonizing took place (200, 500 or 1000 years ago), what the Indigenous circumstances were at the time of colonization, and what geographic or other environmental dynamics contributed to colonization. We will now look at colonization in the U.S., Australia, Canada and Aotearoa/New Zealand for a picture of colonization and its effects. When we do this, we achieve a better understanding of the situation in the U.S. We can also see how it differs from or is similar to the history of Indigenous Peoples in other comparable countries.

Australia, the U.S., Canada and Aotearoa/New Zealand are all developed, wealthy, western, capitalist, democratic countries, but they are geographically separated. All have had Indigenous populations affected by European colonization and all have later become independent. In terms of geography and environment, Australia, Aotearoa/New Zealand, Canada, and the U.S. could not be more different. Colonizing efforts were certainly influenced by, for example, the arctic and subarctic climate of Canada and the largely desert climate of Australia. Aotearoa/New Zealand, with a much smaller landmass compared to the other three countries, present yet another element to consider. The environmental elements were closely interwoven and accommodated within the lives of the Indigenous populations. The details of the colonizing process and the current state of Indigenous affairs and race relations more generally in each of these countries will be explored.

Canada

Canada lies in the northern part of North America, spanning a total area of 9,984,670 square kilometers (CIA, 2020). With a temperate climate in the south, and subarctic and arctic climates in the north, it is perhaps not surprising that 90% of the population lives within 300 miles of the U.S. border. Even so, a number of Indigenous communities reside in the arctic and subarctic regions.

First Nations Peoples have lived in Canada for at least 12,000 years and likely came from Asia and Polynesia. Although there was much trade, early European contact with Indigenous Peoples in what is now called Canada was mainly with the French in the early 1600s. It was peaceful contact mostly related to trade and fishing. Gradually, the British came to the area and, as their interests were in settlement and the land, there were increasingly more conflicts, but these were often between the British and the French. As the British alliances were with different Indigenous groups, it also meant that the conflicts extended into the Indigenous communities.

As is the standard protocol with colonizing efforts, the commonly held date of Canadian colonization is in 1497 when John Cabot landed in Newfoundland, but it wasn't until the 1600s that more permanent settlements were established by the French. The French had a policy of intermarriage between the French and the Indigenous Peoples, which meant that close ties had developed that did not necessarily involve military support or adequate military support against the British. In 1713, France ceded to the British and in 1755, the British 'expelled' all French from the area; the French went south to Louisiana. By 1763, through the Peace of Paris, the French gave up all their claims in the north of North America and in the same year, the Royal Proclamation defined English settlements.

In Canada, the Indian Act of 1876 resulted in land being taken over by the Commonwealth. This meant that Indigenous Peoples lost their traditional livelihoods such as hunting and fishing. Similar to Australia, the Residential School System was put in place in 1892 to 'civilize' the Indigenous children. Children were placed in boarding schools run by churches, where they were not allowed to speak their Indigenous languages and were often abused—physically, sexually and emotionally. It was not until the summer of 2008 that the Canadian Government made an apology to the Indigenous Peoples for the Residential School System and its effects.

The Indigenous Peoples of Canada comprise nearly 4.9% of the total population or 1,670,000 people in 2016 (OECD, 2019). They are generally grouped according to First Nations peoples 60%, Metis 36%, and Inuit 4% (OECD, 2019; see Table 12.1). The Metis population are unique as Indigenous Peoples as they comprise a culture that developed through French and Indigenous intermarriage.

> **Websites**
> For more information about Canada's First Nations and Aboriginal peoples, see the website for Aboriginal Affairs and Northern Development Canada: http://www.aadnc-aandc.gc.ca.
> First Peoples of Canada: http://firstpeoplesofcanada.com.

The United States

Vikings had contact with Indigenous Peoples in North America from as early as the first millennium AD, and European contact was sporadic after that with British, Dutch and French trade. Gradually, roughly between the 1600s and the 1800s, European occupation pushed the Indigenous population westward and the Indigenous Peoples suffered from diseases, genocide, and from being dislocated from their lands. In the late 1800s, reservations were used to contain Indigenous Peoples and, similar to Canadian, Australian and Aotearoa/New Zealand policies at

Table 12.1 Comparison of Indigenous populations and treaty status in four countries

Country	Total Population[1]	Actual size of Indigenous population[2]	Percentage of total population[2]	Indigenous population groupings	Treaties[2]
Australia	25 466 459	798 381	3.3%	Aboriginal (91%) Torres Strait Islander (5%) Both Aboriginal and Torres Strait Islander (4%)[3]	None* Some between individuals, not the British Crown
Canada	37 694 085	1 673 785	4.9%	First Nations (60%) Metis (33%) Inuit (4%) Multiple and other responses (3%)[2]	Treaty status given to those of First Nations heritage who registered with federal government. Health Canada provides free health care to First Nations and Inuit populations who live on reserves and/or Inuit communities. Metis not eligible for treaty status or free health care

(continued)

Table 12.1 (continued)

Country	Total Population[1]	Actual size of Indigenous population[2]	Percentage of total population[2]	Indigenous population groupings	Treaties[2]
Aotearoa/New Zealand	4 925 477	692 300 (Maori ethnic group) 643,977 (Māori descent)	16.3%	Maori (100%)	Treaty of Waitangi (1840) established British control while setting out Maori rights. Treaty is integrated into health policy, with Maori people given rights to partnership, participation and protection in health-related policies
United States	332 639 102	6 706 210	2.0%	American Indian or Alaska Native (AI/AN) only (60%) AI/AN plus another race (40%)	562 federally recognized tribes exist as sovereign entities. U.S. government obligated to provide free health care to federally recognized AI/AN

the time, assimilation processes were well underway. Removing children to boarding schools was common, as was removing elders to rest homes.

Films

See the documentary, *Indian Country Diaries* https://itvs.org/films/indian-country-diaries.

Unspoken: Native American Boarding Schools http://www.pbs.org/video/unspoken-americas-native-american-boarding-schools-oobt1r/.

Native America is a four-part PBS series released in late 2018 http://www.pbs.org/about/blogs/news/pbs-announces-native-america-new-four-part-series-premiering-fall-2018/.

After World War I, 'Indians' became citizens of the U.S. and in the 1950s, moves were made to terminate the reservations programs to fully assimilate the Indigenous Peoples into wider society. As with other countries, during the 1970s policies of 'self-determination' were implemented, though these seem to have been less of a reality than what they appeared on paper. The Indigenous Peoples' reservations were often on land that had little value at the time, but later, some of these lands were found to have oil or other valuable resources. The groups that have been able to keep their reservations have more recently been placed in a compromising position, as valueless land has been seen as a good place for hazardous waste disposal. 'As of 1992, waste disposal interests had approached over fifty reservations to negotiate dumping permits' (Perry, 1996, p. 122).

Today, the U.S. Indigenous population comprises about 2.0% of the total population, but as seen in Table 12.1, it is the largest Indigenous population among those countries compared with about 6.7 million people. The Indigenous population includes many communities, tribes, nations, and bands all across the country, including Alaska, which lies to the far north and to the west of Canada and Hawaii.

Websites

> For more information about the U.S. Indigenous populations, see the Bureau of Indian Affairs website: https://www.bia.gov/.
>
> See the website for the National Congress of American Indians for a wide range of resources including publications, legal findings, testimonies, news, and more: https://www.ncai.org/.

Aotearoa/ New Zealand

The country of Aotearoa/New Zealand includes the North and South islands, together comprising 268,838 square kilometers. The temperate climate is well suited to farming, particularly on the North Island. It is estimated that Māori, the tangata whenua, or people of the land, had been in Aotearoa from before 1300 A.D. The first European contact for Aotearoa/New Zealand Māori was with the Dutch in 1642, but British contact did not occur until 1769 when James Cook arrived. The farming potential of Aotearoa/New Zealand, as well as sealing, whaling, and other trade, attracted European settlers from about the 1790s.

In 1840, the first European settlement in Aotearoa/New Zealand was established in Wellington and the Treaty of Waitangi was signed. The 1840 Treaty of Waitangi served as a contract between the British Crown and Māori, which basically indicated that Māori would retain ownership of their land but that they would recognize British sovereignty. The treaty was written in both English and Māori and there has been some debate about how the treaty was understood by the different parties. The 1975 Waitangi Tribunal was established to help rectify those issues, determining three basic principles to the treaty as partnership, protection, and participation. These principles can theoretically be applied to all situations in Aotearoa/New Zealand. In terms of health, they would require that Māori be active and equal partners in decisions about health, that Māori fully participate in Aotearoa/New Zealand government and society, and that the Aotearoa/New Zealand government take responsibility for protecting Māori interests (for example, ensuring equity).

Māori experience of colonization differed from that in the other countries presented here, particularly as it relates to the signing and honoring of the treaty. Māori of Aotearoa/New Zealand still, however, suffer the negative consequences of colonization, borne out by similar health disparities and intergenerational trauma.

Websites
For more information about Māori in New Zealand see:
   Te Puni Kokiri, the Ministry of Māori Development: http://www.tpk.govt.nz/en/.
   Korero Māori (a resource for Māori Language) http://www.korero.maori.nz/.
   Te Ara for a brief history of Māori: http://www.teara.govt.nz/en/maori.

Film
The 1994 film *Once Were Warriors* is a grueling example of intergenerational trauma that is contextualized within a Māori experience. However, it could just as easily represent any people with similar traumatic histories.
   For another perspective of New Zealand and Māori, readers may enjoy the 2003 film *Whale Rider*.

Australia

Australia comprises 7,741,220 square kilometers, which is slightly smaller than the U.S. contiguous states. The Indigenous Peoples of Australia, the Aboriginal and Torres Strait Islanders, are estimated to have lived in the land currently called Australia for as long as 60,000 years. While trading was occurring between Australia and other places, it was not until 1770 that Captain James Cook laid claim for Great Britain. Dutch contact in Australia occurred in the early 1600 s, it was not until 1788 that Australia was settled by the British for use as a penal colony. Indigenous Australians had trade relations with others long before any European contacts. For example, Indigenous people traded with the Macassan sailors from Indonesia (Trudgen, 2010). In the first 80 years of settlement of Australia, approximately 160,000 people arrived, either as convicts or to support the penal colonies. By 1901, there were nearly four million non-Indigenous people in Australia.

While there were some attempts by early settlers to negotiate land with the Indigenous Peoples, the doctrine of *terra nullius* prevailed until a High Court challenge by Torres Strait Islander Eddie Mabo in 1992 (see the Australian Bureau of Statistics, 1995).

Examples of earlier attempts that appeared to recognize land ownership by Indigenous Peoples are found in the mid-1800s. In 1835, John Batman signed two 'treaties' with Kulin people to 'purchase' 600,000 acres of land between what is now Melbourne and the Bellarine Peninsula. In the same year—in response to these treaties and other arrangements between free settlers and Indigenous inhabitants such as around Camden—the New South Wales governor, Sir Richard Bourke, issued a proclamation. Bourke's proclamation reinforced the notion that the land belonged to no one prior to the British Crown taking possession (Australian Government Culture Portal, n.d.).

More formalized policies impacting on Indigenous Australians were implemented from the 1890s. Generally, the period from the 1890s to the 1950s was considered a time of 'segregation'. This period included ideas of Indigenous Australians needing 'protection', and missions and reserves were established. This was also a time of 'protecting' white Australians from the perceived threat of undesirable or diseased Indigenous people, which was ironic because many diseases that Indigenous Australians suffered were introduced by the early settlers. These various diseases decimated whole family groups and had significant impacts on entire Indigenous populations.

From the 1950s to the 1960s, assimilation policies were implemented. This meant that Indigenous Australians were to merge with mainstream Australia and to erode or eliminate signs of Aboriginality. This period represented Indigenous Peoples as an 'inferior race' that could potentially be 'bred out' through mixing with 'white Australians'.

A relatively brief period from 1967 to 1972 focused on integration, which was meant to be a choice about whether or not to integrate into mainstream Australia. However, children could be refused access to school during this period. Self-determination was only evident from 1972 to 1975, during the Whitlam era. Labor Prime Minister Gough Whitlam initiated many reforms, including the return of land and various forms of Indigenous governance.

Self-management policies were in place from 1975 to 1996, with the Aboriginal and Torres Strait Islander Commission (ATSIC) established in 1988, but by 2004 the commission had been abolished. Reconciliation followed from 1996 to 2007. This period also included a time of 'mutual obligation' and 'new assimilation' under the leadership of former Prime Minister John Howard. Some called these policy directives 'coercive reconciliation', considering the initiatives of the Northern Territory Emergency Response (NTER) (Altman & Hinkson, 2007) which used as an excuse a report into Child Sexual Abuse to introduce a range of draconian and punitive measures against Indigenous Australians. The effects of this response are still being felt today, with Indigenous people, men in particular, vilified as potential perpetrators and whole communities stigmatized and further disempowered.

There are many events implicated in the health and well-being of people today. This is a very brief overview of some of the policies affecting Indigenous Australians. For more details, see for example, Eckermann et al. (2010) or look at the Australian Law Reform Commission (2010b).

Some Comparisons

Many other peoples around the world were colonized by other groups and nations and often the colonizing of a land required the enslavement of Africans and Indigenous Peoples in order to survive. Have a look at some of the areas colonized by the French, for example. How did these experiences differ?

The estimated length of time that Indigenous Peoples inhabited different continents varies widely between continents. Some evidence suggests that Indigenous Peoples inhabited Australia for as long as 60,000 years. While there is some debate around how long Māori have lived in Aotearoa/New Zealand and exactly where the Māori people originally came from, the estimated time of occupation is believed to be around 1,200 years. In the present day U.S. and Canada, there is evidence of Indigenous villages that date back to the 700s. All of the countries were colonized by Europeans from around the late 1700s to the early 1800s. Independence from Britain was in 1776 in the U.S., 1852 for Aotearoa/New Zealand, and 1901 for Australia. However, this independence from the colonizers did not translate into independence in the same way for Indigenous Peoples as it did for others. For example, in Australia, it took another 63 years before Indigenous Australians were given the right to vote. In the U.S., Native Americans were not accepted as citizens until 1924.

Assimilation was a common policy in many countries, requiring that Indigenous Peoples not speak their own languages and not practice traditions or ceremonies—that they become like the 'settler' population. This has had devastating effects internationally, although there is some progress to be seen in the recovery from this damage. For example, in some Māori communities, around 40% of the people speak their tribal language with increasing percentages of young people being able to do so. In North America, there are about 175 languages remaining of the estimated 300 original languages (McMaster & Trafzer, 2008). However, in Australia, there are less than 100 languages from the nearly 300 languages that were spoken when Australia was colonized. Similarly, in the U.S., there were estimated to be around 300 Native languages prior to colonization but today there are only 167 Native languages still in use.

An interesting difference between Australian and Aotearoa/New Zealand Indigenous Peoples and those in the Americas is land boundaries. Australia and Aotearoa/New Zealand have their boundaries defined through being surrounded by water. However, in the Americas, particularly in North and Central America, boundaries have been defined politically through colonization and have overridden Indigenous nation boundaries. Within Australia, the same has happened with state and territory boundaries. That is, colonization has overridden Indigenous nation boundaries. When Indigenous nation boundaries cross later-derived 'state' boundaries, it causes financial and resource implications for many who are accessing health services within their own Indigenous nation boundaries. For example, renal patients from remote Central Australia are at times subject to the rigidity of imposed state and territory borders that determine their access to renal services. Can you identify any similarities in the U.S?

'How Indigenous Are You?'

Indigenous Peoples globally have had their indigeneity questioned and measured, with differing implications for access to resources and impacts on people. For example, in Canada, Indigenous status was determined through groups of people having treaty arrangements with the government. What this meant was that if a group did not have a treaty arrangement, then that group essentially did not exist as 'Indigenous'. Undercounting the Indigenous population has been one strategy of governments to justify inaction or making the Indigenous population 'invisible'.

In the U.S., contention over Indigenous status goes both ways, with huge diversity in the rules about who can and cannot be considered Indigenous and therefore have access or not to certain benefits. Indeed, some groups have even resorted to 'tribal disenrollment' (Wilson & Yellow Bird, 2005). While disenrollment may be related to genuine concern about people inappropriately accessing and using services intended for Indigenous Peoples, others suggest that it is based on greed and that this greed results in loss of services such as schooling and health care for those who need those services (Wilson & Yellow Bird, 2005). This illustrates that Indigenous status and access to resources is not a simple issue, but certainly a global one.

Terminology

As discussed earlier in this text, the terminology used to describe Indigenous Peoples, or any group for that matter, is critically important. In considering the global context of Indigenous issues, we see again the diversity of peoples and how, in each country, Indigenous Peoples may be identified or identify themselves. In Aotearoa/New Zealand, the Indigenous Peoples are Māori, with many different *iwi* (tribal groups). Generally, Māori would never be referred to as 'Aboriginal'. In Australia, as discussed, the terms 'Aboriginal Peoples' and 'Torres Strait Island Peoples' are used, and it is common to also use the term 'Indigenous' when talking about the general Indigenous Australian population (but remember that these terms are not universally accepted in Australia). Not all Indigenous Peoples in Australia are either Aboriginal or Torres Strait Islanders. For example, there are people known as Kanakas who are the descendants of people forcibly brought to Australia in a shameful process known as 'blackbirding'—which was basically akin to what happened to people from Africa who were forcibly enslaved. People from various Pacific Islands like Vanuatu were tricked or coerced onto ships and brought to Queensland to work as 'indentured servants' in the sugar cane industry. It is believed there may be as many as 20,000 descendants living in Queensland today.

Reading
See the ABC news website for an article from 16 August 2013: 'Calls for an official apology over 'blackbirding' trade on 150th anniversary': http://www.abc.net.au/news/2013-08-14/an-blackbirding-special/4887692.

In Canada, the Indigenous Peoples are also referred to as 'Aboriginal', but the main groupings are First Nations (or First Peoples), Inuit, and Metis. Again, there are many subgroups and nations, communities, or tribes. In the U.S., the Indigenous Peoples are often referred to as 'Indians' or 'American Indians' or 'Native Americans', though some of these terms can be contentious due to their history. When the first explorers went to *Great Turtle Island* what is now the U.S., they thought that they were at the Indian subcontinent and so called the people 'Indians'. For that reason, some people prefer to use 'Native' or 'Native Americans' to describe the Indigenous Peoples of the U.S. Note, however, that the term 'Native' may be seen as offensive in Australia or Aotearoa/New Zealand. The U.S., as a nation, includes the state of Alaska, in the far northwest of Canada. The Indigenous Peoples there are often referred to as 'Alaska Native' and are a good example of the previous discussion about imposed national boundaries overriding Indigenous boundaries. Overall, the populations are highly diverse, and people were often forced to live together on 'reservations'. It was assumed that this would be appropriate, and this practice failed to recognize that maybe everyone who was being forced to live together wouldn't get along. Overall, it is important to remember the diversity of Indigenous Peoples and to be respectful of how people choose to identify themselves, regardless of government-imposed labels or categories.

In New Zealand the concept of *ethnicity* is self-determined. That is, ethnicity relates to the cultural groups to which you consider yourself belonging. It is not determined by someone else. So someone may consider themselves to ethnically identify with a particular group, but not by descent or ancestry. This could arise, for example, through adoption, community involvement, or marriage. In contrast, the criteria for Indigenous identity in Australia is:

1. being of Aboriginal or Torres Strait Islander descent
2. self-identification as Aboriginal or Torres Strait Islander
3. being accepted as such by the community they live in or have lived in (ALRC, 2010a).

There are a few concerns with these criteria and the way that 'ethnicity' is measured in general in Australia. Ethnicity is not directly classified in the Australian census; rather, a range of variables can be used to imply ethnicity. These include country of birth, country of parents' birth, language indicators (such as language spoken at home or proficiency in English), religious affiliation, and year of arrival in Australia. The most direct questions relating to ethnicity in the Australian census are, 'what is the person's ancestry' and, for Aboriginal and Torres Strait Islanders, 'is the person of Aboriginal or Torres Strait Islander origin?' As a comparison, in New Zealand, individuals are asked, 'what country were you born in?', 'which ethnic group do you belong to?', and a series of questions relating to Māori descent and tribal (*iwi*) affiliations and *iwi* area (*rohe*).

> **Critical Thinking**
> How can we learn from identity questions used in other countries?
> How do these differing ways of measuring identity influence how we think about identity as a nation and what are the consequences of these differing ways of measuring identity?

Disease and Colonization

A common feature of colonization was that the colonizers often brought with them diseases that had devastating effects on Indigenous populations. Without ever having been exposed to these new diseases and with little immunity, it was not difficult for an illness that had moderate effects on the settlers to kill entire families and large numbers of Indigenous populations in whole communities. For example, in Canada, 'the Huron also lost over half of their population in a measles epidemic between 1634 and 1640' (Perry, 1996, p. 127). Other tribal groups, such as the Iroquois, were also affected. For a more malicious example, intentional attempts to infect Indigenous Peoples with deadly illnesses were seen at Fort Pitt when two blankets and a handkerchief infected with smallpox were 'gifted' to members of the Delaware who came to persuade the British to abandon their fort (Fenn, 2000).

The Most Recent Contacts

In Australia, there are Aboriginal people alive today who could tell you about when they first met the first 'white' people. Such recency of contact is unique to Australia as a developed country. For some Central Australian and Western Desert peoples, contact with these new people happened as recently as 1970. Indeed, the last remaining family group to enter settlements in the Western Desert came in the mid-1980s, not because they were 'lost' as the media portrayed them, but due to drought conditions and the fact that all their relatives had since moved into life in the settlements. Vast distances, lack of transport infrastructure (such as paved roads), and cost, means that life, particularly in remote desert communities, is very different from that in the coastal urban centers of Australia.

The relatively smaller land mass of Aotearoa/New Zealand means that distance did not present the same issues, although a different sort of challenging terrain has access implications. Canada, on the other hand, with an arctic and subarctic climate in the north and separation of land by water, presents yet other dynamics to the colonization of land and people. The very cold weather meant that only the most southern parts of Canada were useable for farming. Hence, the northern areas were of less interest to the British and others, so Indigenous Peoples in the northern areas were less or differently affected by colonizing efforts.

When we consider that for some people, 'contact' with white, western, European culture, either through the domination of land and people or enslavement, has occurred within living memory, the notions that 'it's all in the past' and that people need to 'just get over it' are seriously flawed and hurtful to those affected by such rapid change. From another perspective, the last survivor of the transatlantic 'slave trade', Matilda McCrear, died in just 1940 (Coughlan, 2020).

Population and Health Status of Indigenous Peoples in a Global context

Table 12.1 provides a comparison of the Indigenous populations and treaties in Australia, Canada, Aotearoa/New Zealand, and the U.S. There are always various limitations to the data used, especially when those data are being compared across many different countries. Even so, it is useful to attempt to make the comparisons. They show us how other countries collect and analyze data and give us ideas about how to improve our data (see AIHW, 2011).

Overall, Table 12.1 shows that, in numbers, the Indigenous population in the U.S. is the largest, followed by Canada, and Australia's Indigenous population is not much smaller than Aotearoa/New Zealand's. As a percentage of the country's total population, however, we see that Aotearoa/New Zealand has the highest proportion of Indigenous Peoples (16%), followed by Canada (4.9%), then Australia (3.3%) and the U.S. (2.0%). Most of the countries described have between two and four official Indigenous population groupings, although the category of 'Māori' is used in Aotearoa/New Zealand. However, as discussed previously, there is much diversity in the Indigenous groups in each of these countries and these categories often do not adequately reflect that diversity. Table 12.1 also shows that Australia is the only country that does not have a treaty with the Indigenous Peoples. Indeed, this is often cited as a major failure of Australia and a major contributor to the overall poor health and social status of Indigenous Australians today.

Can We Fix Our Problems by Doing What Others Do?

It can be very useful to see what other countries are doing in terms of Indigenous issues or Indigenous health in particular. However, we must be very mindful of how 'transplanting' programs, ideas, or approaches can potentially serve to undermine local Indigenous knowledge, ideas, and capacity. On the other hand, it can be useful to look at programs, ideas, and policies from other locations and countries. Doing so can save time and effort—we do not always need to 'reinvent the wheel'. Overall, it is essential that programs or approaches be developed in consultation and true partnership and participation with the people involved or those who will be affected by whatever is being proposed. Ideas from other countries might help to serve as a basis for discussion, but these can then be adapted or modified to suit the purposes, issues, or unique social and cultural dynamics of the particular group involved. Within the U.S., a program or policy may be developed in one state or with one community, but it may not necessarily work, or be appropriate, in another state or with another community. Cultural safety, for example, cannot simply be transplanted to the U.S. setting without consideration of some key differences in history, experiences of colonization, demography, geography, politics, and cultures.

Decolonization and Health and Human Service Professionals

If we accept that 'colonization' is much more than moving in and setting up a place to live, that it involves a gradual and often subtle erosion of people's lives, then '*de*colonization' necessarily involves more than just land rights and politics. Colonization is often seen as the *direct* cause of the health and social conditions affecting Indigenous Peoples globally, which is why it is so important that *decolonization* is essential to solving health and social problems (Edwards & Taylor, 2008). *Decolonization* has been defined as 'the intelligent, calculated, and active resistance to the forces of colonialism that perpetuate the subjugation and/or exploitation of our minds, bodies, and lands, and it is engaged for the ultimate purpose of overturning the colonial structure and realizing Indigenous liberation' (Wilson & Yellow Bird, 2005, p. 2). From Aotearoa/New Zealand, decolonization has been discussed as below:

> The processes of decolonisation are not universal. Where there are clearly commonalities, there are also specifics that need to be identified as a part of the overall decolonisation agenda. Our colonial experience has been

one of denial. Denial of our reo [language], denial of our tikanga [cultural practices], denial of our whenua [land], denial of our taonga [treasures], denial of our whakapapa [genealogy]. Colonial forces have attempted to deny us all of those things that contribute to our notions of who we are and where we fit in the world. The ways in which these attempts were made varied dependent on context and location, as such the effects have been diverse and multilayered. Decolonisation then includes a peeling back of the layers. Layer by layer. Constantly reflecting on what we find (Pihama Pihama, 2001, *sic*).

Decolonizing is an important process for everyone. Decolonizing practice for health and human services professionals includes practicing the many concepts that have been discussed throughout this text. It is about not disempowering, diminishing, or demeaning those in your care or those with whom you work. It is about being regardful of the history that has affected people and not perpetuating the damaging colonizing efforts. Being respectful and encouraging people's use of their own languages and not denying them their right to speak their own language is also part of 'decolonizing' your practice. Challenging the hierarchical nature of healthcare practice and services even helps to decolonize health services and practice.

> **Critical Thinking**
> Read the passage below. It was written about the Aboriginal situation in Canada but may well have been written about the U.S., Australia or Aotearoa/New Zealand or many other colonized countries. Consider how misunderstandings in healthcare or human services still happen today. Fundamental misunderstandings, as illustrated in the below passage, could easily be replicated in a health situation today—for example, when there is not a shared understanding of illness or treatment.
>
>> Although from the government's perspective, treaties had become a matter of extinguishing indigenous claims, in the view of many indigenous people, the treaties continued to be agreements establishing formal relationships with the government. In many cases, indigenous groups interpreted them as promises of friendship or protection from further encroachment.

> Although indigenous peoples had no doubts about their inherent rights to the territories under agreement, they generally did not share European concepts of absolute ownership. Many had long-established views of group territory, but usually these involved communal or conventionally agreed-upon access to natural resources. The idea of selling lands as if they were private property made little sense to them. In most cases, it seems, they saw treaties as devices for establishing relationships between people rather than between people and land.
>
> Many viewed the treaty process in terms of social or political agreements rather than economic transactions, as agreements to allow others to use the land they had occupied. But they did not necessarily accept the interpretation that they, themselves, could not continue to hunt there or use it in other ways. They tended to interpret the payments they received as 'presents' or gifts, tokens of agreement—that is, expressions of social ties—rather than as compensation for relinquishing their lands to others forever [sic] (Perry, 1996, p. 134).

Activity
- Discuss any differences in the experiences, responses, or consequences of colonization.
- What difference, if any, have treaties made to the health and wel-lbeing of Indigenous Peoples? What is your view on treaties with Indigenous Peoples in the U.S.?
- Define and describe what might be required of health or human services professionals in undertaking a process of decolonization as required by the cultural safety proponents. What might this mean in a day-to-day practice sense?

Conclusion

We have discussed the histories and the health statuses of Indigenous Peoples in the U.S., Canada, Aotearoa/New Zealand, and Australia. We have discussed similarities and differences, but overall, explored the detrimental effects of colonizing histories. We can see that the strategies of colonization have resulted in similar detrimental health outcomes in countries geographically separated.

Overall, we have seen a number of similarities and differences between the colonizing histories of Australia, the U.S., Canada, and Aotearoa/New Zealand. Acknowledging these colonizing histories and how these histories continue to harm health and well-being today is one step toward healing and safety for everyone.

References

Altman, J., & Hinkson, M. (Eds.). (2007). *Coercive Reconciliation: Stabilise, normalise, exit Aboriginal Australia*. Arena Publications Association.

Australian Bureau of Statistics (ABS). (1995). Year Book Australia, 1995, 1301.0, The Mabo Case and the Native Title Act. www.abs.gov.au/Ausstats/abs@.nsf/Previousproducts/1301.0Feature%20Article21995.

Australian Government Culture Portal. (n.d.). *European discovery and the colonisation of Australia*, Australian Government Culture Portal. www.cultureandrecreation.gov.au/articles/australianhistory/index.htm.

AIHW (Australian Institute of Health and Welfare). (2011). *Comparing life expectancy of Indigenous people in Australia, New Zealand, Canada and the United States: Conceptual, methodological and data issues*. https://www.aihw.gov.au/report/comparing-life-expectancy-of-indigenous-people-in-australia-new-zealand-canada-and-the-united-states-conceptual-methodological-and-data-issues/formats.

ALRC (Australian Law Reform Commission). (2010a). Essentially yours: The protection of human genetic information in Australia (ALRC Report 96)/36. Kinship and Identity, Legal Definitions of Aboriginality. http://www.alrc.gov.au/publications/36-kinship-and-identity/legal-definitions-aboriginality.

ALRC (Australian Law Reform Commission). (2010b). Chapter 3 'Aboriginal Societies: The experience of contact: Changing policies toward Aboriginal people'. www.alrc.gov.au/publications/3.%20Aboriginal%20Societies%3A%20The%20Experience%20of%20Contact/changing-policies-towards-aboriginal.

CIA. (2020). *The World Factbook*. https://www.cia.gov/the-world-factbook/.

Coughlan, S. (2020, March 25). Last survivor of Atlantic Slave Trade discovered. *BBC*. https://www.bbc.com/news/education-52010859.

Eckermann, A., Dowd, T., Nixon, L., Chong, E., Gray, R., & Johnson, S. (2010). *Binah Goonj: Bridging cultures in Aboriginal health*. Churchill Livingstone Elsevier.

Edwards, T., & Taylor, K. (2008). Decolonising cultural awareness. *Australian Nursing Journal*. Australian Nursing Federation.

Fenn, E. (2000). Biological warfare in eighteenth-century North America: Beyond Jeffery Amherst. *The Journal of American History, 86*(4), 1552–1580. https://doi.org/10.2307/2567577, https://www.jstor.org/stable/2567577?seq=1.

McMaster, G., & Trafzer, C. E. (Eds.). (2008). *Native Universe: Voices of Indian America* (*Native American Tribal Leaders, Writers, Scholars, and Story Tellers*). National Museum of the American Indian. Smithsonian Institution in association with *National Geographic*.

Migration Policy Institute. (n.d.). Comparing Migrant Stock: The Foreign Born in Australia, Canada, and the United States by Region of Origin. https://www.migrationpolicy.org/programs/data-hub/comparing-migrant-stock-foreign-born-australia-canada-and-united-states-region.

OECD. (2019). *Linking Indigenous Communities with Regional Development*. http://www.oecd.org/publications/linking-indigenous-communities-with-regional-development-3203c082-en.htm.

Perry, R. J. (1996). *From time immemorial: Indigenous peoples and state systems*. University of Texas Press.

Pihama Pihama, L. (2001). *Mana Wahine*, unpublished PhD thesis. Auckland University.

Trudgen, R. (2010). *Why warriors lie down and die*. Aboriginal Resource and Development Services Inc., Darwin.

Wilson, W.A. and Yellow Bird, M. (eds). (2005). 'Beginning decolonization'. In *For Indigenous Eyes Only: A decolonization handbook*, School of American Research.

World Health Organization. (2007). *Health of Indigenous peoples Fact sheet* N°326 October. https://www.who.int/gender-equity-rights/knowledge/factsheet-indigenous-healthn-nov2007-eng.pdf?ua=1.

13

Reflection as a Tool of Culturally Safe Practice

Reflection is a powerful tool for learning, development, and growth and is a key component of culturally safe practice. Through reflection, in and on practice, health professionals have an opportunity to examine their interactions with the goal of providing culturally safe and effective care.

This chapter describes reflective practice and how it relates to improving outcomes for all clients. We especially focus on those who experience the greatest disparities and anyone who differs from the dominant culture of the health and human services and providers. Reflection is applied to help health and human service professionals to decolonize and move toward culturally safe practice. Finally, we examine the relevance of this topic to your practice, and the transferability of reflective practice that is regardful in any setting.

Chapter Objectives

After completing this chapter, you should be able to:

- understand the concept of reflective practice
- identify principles and strategies for reflecting on and within practice
- reflect on the role of individual health professionals in cultural safety at an organizational level
- consider ongoing developments in cultural safety.

Reflection

Reflection on practice is not only a key principle of cultural safety, but also a requisite competency in a number of health and social service professions. There are many strategies that can be used for reflection, from simple sharing of work-related stories with colleagues or friends to more structured approaches such as keeping a professional journal or participating in formal debriefing with colleagues or supervisors.

In a cultural safety context, reflection requires some critique and understanding of one's own culture and how it might influence our interactions with someone who may be of a different cultural background. Importantly when you use reflection as a tool, it should not be limited to simply thinking about and being aware—it then needs application in professional practice.

Do you know your own culture well enough to recognize where it might impact on your interactions with someone? We asked earlier for readers to reflect on how they felt about certain cultural values and norms. You might appreciate that no one has been asked in this book to change what you believe or feel (although that may happen as interactions with those who are not the same as ourselves challenge our existing beliefs and attitudes). What is required to enact cultural safety in practice is to be able to acknowledge what your possible biases, assumptions, stereotypes, or judgments are that we all bring to an encounter. We then need to make sure that these do not harm the person we are providing care or service to through our actions.

Rather than being fearful of making mistakes, or of not knowing something, reflective practice offers the opportunity to stop, consider, and try again if necessary. The point is that cultural values can profoundly influence the judgments, attitudes, and responses to the observed behaviors and practices of people from a differing cultural background and unless you consciously take notice, interactions that are intended to help can have harmful consequences.

What Is Reflective Practice?

Reflective practice is knowing that you do not know it all, and that what you have learned as a student through formal education is not the end of your education but is part of a career-long, even lifelong, process. Through reflection on your practice, acknowledging and exploring your knowledge or lack of knowledge, your discomforts, the ways you interact with others and the strategies you employ to remedy issues, your practice can be improved (Bulman & Shutz, 2004). Bassot (2016) adds that a genuinely reflective approach requires an engagement with your feelings and the need to question your assumptions.

Johns and Freshwater (2005) look at the different layers of reflection, which provides a useful framework for how to engage in reflective practice. These include reflection-on-experience, reflection-in-action, the internal supervisor, reflection-within-the-moment, and mindful practice. These are explained more in Table 13.1.

> **Activity**
> Choose an experience you may have had or witnessed where a cultural difference was significant such as gender, ability, ethnicity, or other difference. Use John's (2017) Reflection on Action to draw 'insights that may inform future practice in positive ways'. In other words, what can you learn from your reflection on this experience?
> - What principles of cultural safety were absent or evident?
> - What could have been done differently?

Table 13.1 Layers of reflection (adapted from Johns, 2017)

Reflection element	Description
Reflection on experience	Reflecting on a situation or experience after the event with the intention of drawing insights that may inform future practice in positive ways
Reflection in action	Pausing within a particular situation or experience in order to make sense and reframe the situation so as to be able to proceed towards desired outcomes
The internal supervisor	Dialoguing with self while in conversation with another in order to make sense
Reflection within the moment	Being aware of thinking, feeling, and responding within the unfolding moment and dialoguing with self to ensure interpretation and responses are congruent to whatever is unfolding. It is having some space in your mind to change your ideas rather than being fixed on certain ideas
Mindful practice	Being aware of self within the unfolding moment with the intention of realizing desirable practice (however 'desirable' is known)

- What potential harms or benefits could you identify from the experience?
- Have you used any of the other layers of reflection? If so, which ones and what insights did you gain?

Schön (1983) discusses the differences between reflection-in-action and reflection-on-action. Reflection-in-action is when we think about what we are doing while we are doing it, whereas reflection-on-action is when we later think about something we did earlier. In terms of practice, reflection-in-action might be noticing while you are doing it that you have had a joke or a moment of connection with a client or that something you said seemed to get a client thinking about an issue. Reflection-on-action might be taking the time, at the end of the day, to review the clients you had, how you handled various situations, the conflicts that arose, and how you managed them. Sometimes it is only when reflecting back on a situation that you get an 'aha' moment—perhaps in a situation you were not quite sure what a client was trying to say, but later, when reflecting on the situation, it 'clicked': 'aha! *Now I know what they were trying to say!*'.

In terms of cultural safety, the ideas of reflection, as presented by theorists Freire (1972) and Mezirow (1991) are particularly relevant (as cited in McEldowney et al., 2006). Specifically, Freire proposed the idea of 'praxis', which relates to the values that inform practice and considers the function of social justice in health care (McEldowney et al., 2006). Freire also wrote about 'conscientization', or having a consciousness about practice. Mezirow, on the other hand, felt that reflection was much greater than simply thinking about what we are doing, but involves thinking about our relationships, the organizational structures that we work within and the larger social and political influences on what we do.

In terms of health, the complexities can become almost overwhelming. In order to cope, practitioners might just 'do their job' without reflecting on practice, and in the process unfortunately become desensitized to the issues. If we take Mezirow's concept of reflection that involves relationships, organizational structures, and social and political influences, as we have shown throughout this book, health is complex indeed. Relationships may be challenged as professionals learn new ways to communicate and interact with others and organizational structures may further constrain working effectively with clients. For example, access and appropriateness of services may be less than ideal and the health professional may find that there is little they can do to change it. This was demonstrated in research by Grant and Guerin (2018) where they found that child and family health nurses struggled to provide culturally safe care when it conflicted with policies. As a health or human services professional, you may find yourself in politically motivated situations in which reflection may be necessary to examine whether your actions are aiming for cultural safety or perpetuating unsafe service or care for people who differ from yourself.

According to Oelke et al. (2013, p. 369), 'Cultural safety focuses on relationship and social justice with a critical analysis of historical, political and social knowledge of individuals and institutions. Critical reflection is essential to facilitate professionals' discovery of new meaning or reconstructing existing meaning (Browne et al., 2009) enabling culturally safe care for individuals and communities'. Bassot (2016) also highlights the importance for reflective practice to be 'critical' and underpinned by 'reflexivity'. Being 'critical' in this sense is not about criticizing but being analytical or constructively assessing something. Reflexivity involves mindfulness and being aware of what we think, feel, and how we are acting and being aware of the assumptions that we make (Bassot, 2016). Howatson-Jones (2016) defines reflexivity as 'reflecting on the specifics of situations, as well as the conditions from which they arise, and how we might be implicated in those conditions' (p. 85). Critically reflective practice takes simple reflection a step further to examine power relationships in health care practice and how that power can be misused and can lead to discriminatory and even oppressive practice (Bassot, 2016).

Cultural safety is an ongoing, continually re-assessable aspiration. It's only when the client deems that your care is 'safe' that you can say you have achieved it—for that client, in that situation. The important thing with reflection is that it be used as a tool to improve practice, rather than to criticize anyone for not getting it right every time. It is only through reflection that improvements can be made to practice. Cultural safety is not about feeling terrible for our mistakes and misreading of situations, unless of course those things are done without regard or care for others or done with deliberate discrimination.

Activity
- Think of a situation where you may not have handled something as well as you would have liked. What was the situation? What were the consequences of not getting it right?
- Try to do this activity with a friend and see what their reflections might be.
- There are numerous models for reflection and analysis, and we have only mentioned a few. Find a model that you can use to reflect upon the situation for elements of cultural safety.

While reflective practice can be done at a personal, individual level, developing reflective practice among groups and encouraging reflective practice among supervisors and management is also necessary to fully achieve the benefits possible (Bassot, 2016).

Much of what we have talked about through this book has focused on what professionals might do in practice to ensure cultural safety for their clients. Some of the changes needed may be relatively small and easy to apply and some may seem way beyond 'the pay grade'. But in choosing to enter the 'service' professions, you have probably already recognized that health and social care is more than the individual engagements we have with clients. It's history, politics, social justice, economics, and more.

Cultural safety began when an Indigenous midwifery student stood up in a workshop and challenged the facilitators to consider that health and well-being was more than clinical safety (Ramsden, 2002; Wepa, 2015). That is the power of an individual. That brave question set in motion the development of a transformative way of working that has gone around the world. And like all theories and philosophies, others have since critiqued it, argued about it, embraced it, and refined or adapted it to a range of contexts.

Curtis, et al. (2019) suggest that cultural safety should now be redefined to achieve health equity. They recommend an approach to cultural safety that encompasses the following core principles:

- Be clearly focused on achieving health equity, with measurable progress toward this endpoint;
- Be centered on clarified concepts of cultural safety and critical consciousness rather than narrow based notions of cultural competency;
- Be focused on the application of cultural safety within a healthcare systemic/organizational context in addition to the individual health provider-patient interface;
- Focus on cultural safety activities that extend beyond acquiring knowledge about 'other cultures' and developing appropriate skills and attitudes and move to interventions that acknowledge and address biases and stereotypes;

- Promote the framing of cultural safety as requiring a focus on power relationships and inequities within health care interactions that reflect historical and social dynamics.
- Not be limited to formal training curricula but be aligned across all training/practice environments, systems, structures, and policies (Curtis et al., 2019, p. 14).

Cultural Safety Principles for Practice: An Opportunity to Reflect

Throughout this book, we have presented some of the key principles of cultural safety that we have found to be useful when working with clients. Indeed, the following practice principles are relevant to your practice in general, with anyone who you are working with. We have explored these in some previous chapters, but it is worth revisiting them and considering them in the context of reflective practice.

The first principle, to provide care that is *regardful* of culture, directly challenges the status quo of providing care *regardless* of culture. Treating all clients the same, regardless of culture, fails to acknowledge the unique needs and issues affecting people who are culturally different, either to one another or to the professional. Users of health or human services should not have to jettison their cultural values and preferred ways of doing things in order to receive care. Of course, there is the option of exercising choice and going to a culturally specific service. However, all citizens are entitled to an equal opportunity to achieve optimal health; this does not mean necessarily by sameness.

> **Critical Thinking**
> How do you feel now about the idea of treating people the same? Has anything changed for you after exploring this notion of being regardful or different rather than regardless? If you remain unconvinced by the arguments in this book, write down your reasons. Provide rationales for your answers, not your opinion or feelings.

The second principle, to *engage in dialogue*, sounds like a simple thing to do, but even where there is no language barrier, cultural and other communication barriers make this challenging in practice.

> **Scenario**
> A single father has been in small rural hospital for a few days with his sick child. He often leaves during the day and the child is naturally distressed and cries for her father. Another mother sharing the room is looking after her sick child. She sits by the bed all day and tries to organize her family through phone calls and through visitors coming to see the mother and child. Meals are served in the afternoon and by the time the father comes back his meal has been taken away.
>
> 'No, you're too late. You missed your dinner' says the nurse, when he asked if there was any food left. Later in the evening the same nurse quietly asks the woman sharing the room if she would like a cup of coffee and something more to eat. They chat cheerfully about how early the meals are served. The nurse then suggests that the mom take a break and go home for a few hours, reassuring her that the child will be ok. The father on the other side of the curtain is not offered any such support.
>
> - What might be behind these differing responses from the health professional?
> - What assumptions have been made?
> - Why was there no apparent dialogue with the father who left during the day?
> - Why does one parent elicit empathy and compassion and the other does not?
> - How aware or unaware might each be of the dynamics being played out?
> - Describe the power relationships in this scenario.
> - What questions and issues would you like to have discussed with both parents?
> - Turn your reflection to the organization. What responsibility does the health service have for the experience of the client who kept leaving?
> - How might the environment have been made more culturally safe? What supports, personnel or resources would have been helpful in the situation described?

The third principle of culturally safe practice is to be mindful of *whose values are being valued*. Generally, our values are unstated or assumed, and we do not tend to think about our values until they have been challenged. However, our values can have significant impacts on client care, so much so that competency standards include a number of references to values. They also ensure that values are not imposed on clients and that client values if in conflict with those of the health professional, do not compromise the client's care and are respected. Values, however, are an abstract concept and there can be a very fine line between respecting another's values and compromising their care. Interpretation of values is not easy, which is also why reflection is important. For example, you might know someone, or maybe you yourself, who does not put high value on having an immaculately clean and tidy house. Nevertheless, at what point is an unclean or untidy house a health hazard? Of course, it can become a health risk, but there are many degrees to such a judgment. This is a good example of a value, how it can be imposed and how a value can be expressed in different ways.

A child not wearing shoes might, in some settings, be interpreted as not being cared for properly or even neglected. However, in other contexts, not wearing shoes might be perfectly acceptable. We are not suggesting here that 'differing values' should be an excuse for inaction when that may well be called for. There can be a very fine line between value differences and neglect. However, in such an instance, it is critical to engage the relevant people themselves in establishing whether something is culturally appropriate or whether it is an example of dysfunction.

Another principle of cultural safety is to *examine power* in practice and work to minimize inequalities between yourself and the clients. The power of the professional is often not acknowledged in practice, but it can affect care and practice, both on the part of the health professional as well as on the part of the client. For example, a professional has power in terms of medical knowledge, and power in terms of negotiating treatments and services. You as an individual may not feel powerful, but relative to your clients or other workers in your team, you can be more or less powerful at different points.

13 Reflection as a Tool of Culturally Safe Practice

Page and Meerabeau (cited in Elliot, 2004) believe that if the reflector perceives themselves to be in a powerless position to orchestrate changes or suffers from professional apathy, learning and practice are unlikely to be advanced. Thus, successful reflection is as much about the attitude of the clinician as the topic or theme being explored.

> **Scenario**
> A man was discussing treatment options for his failing kidneys. He was a non-drinker and because he had young children, he naturally wanted to be around for them. They discussed dialysis which would have been really difficult as he came from a rural area and would have had to relocate to access services. He asked his doctor about the potential of a kidney transplant, but the doctor advised that this was not an option. Other staff who were present later asked the doctor what the barriers were to this client being considered for a transplant. They knew the man to be strongly committed to his treatment. They were told that the client was 'unlikely to comply with the medication regime' and was unlikely to be able to comply with the strict transplant requirements.
> - It's too obvious to ask who here had the power, but what message does this send about the value of this man to society?
> - What role might the other staff have in advocating for this patient?
> - Who should have been involved in the decision-making?
>
> Revisit the scenario above about the two parents. What values were being privileged in the scenario? What does a 'good' parent do when their child is sick? They often stay vigilant by the child's side, stoically resisting all offers to leave, because the core value for being a 'good parent' for some people is demonstrated in this way. For the single father that left during the day, his core values may have caused him to choose to leave the child in the capable hands of the hospital staff while they did the 'good parent' thing of attending to the rest of the family's needs.
>
> Instead, assumptions are made by all concerned, including the clients, without actually engaging in dialogue. Judgments, lack of empathy, and misuse of power—either consciously or unconsciously—ensure that the experience of health care is very different for both families.
>
> You might have realized by now that in most of the scenarios presented in this text, we have frequently not specified race or ethnicity, gender,

> age, or other possible cultural identities. Did you notice any previously unrealized assumptions, stereotypes, or biases of your own that led you to apply a racial or ethnic, gender, age, sexual orientation, or other backgrounds to the characters while thinking through the questions? Were any receptionists male in your vision of these scenarios? If not, why not? Being able to reflect is the most effective way to check your assumptions and possible biases.

The principle that *process is more important than outcomes* is an interesting one. Research shows that good process results in better outcomes, but if we focus on outcomes exclusively, the process is often compromised, and the outcomes are poorer. Do you think that clients are more interested in having a provider who is highly knowledgeable or one who cares about them? We would hope to provide both, but some research shows that clients are more interested in being cared about (Frankel & Stein, 1999). This links back to the discussion above on empathy. It does not take much longer to show compassion and concern to a client, but it can make a big difference to the outcomes of the care. The process of care also involves more than just any individual health professional along the path.

Think about access to care and services—can clients access the care or services readily? Are there transport or other costs associated with accessing the care that need to be considered? If medication has been prescribed, have any barriers to accessing the medication or taking it been explored? For example, has the cost of the medication been considered and addressed? If the medication has to be refrigerated or if it needs to be taken at certain times (such as with food), has this been addressed? What about the reception staff—have they done all that they could do to reduce barriers to accessing the service? Who should receive cultural safety training in health services?

You might intend to provide culturally safe care for your client but if their experience is an unsafe one at the front door, your efforts could be thwarted. Curtis et al. (2019), suggest widening the cultural safety training for staff and curricula to ensure organizations and systems are prepared for the job.

We discussed racism and discrimination and noted that a key element here is not what someone's intentions might be, but rather, how someone might experience a situation or an interaction. As a culturally safe professional, reflect on policies, practices, and procedures in your workplace as well as your own interactions. Can you identify discriminatory practices in your workplace or somewhere you have attended? How might it be changed to reduce that possibility?

Become more aware of how your own interactions and the workplace environment can be colonizing and consider the ways that you might begin to decolonize your practice. Colonizing practices can be revealed through how language is used or the assumptions that are made. What behaviors could contribute to continuing to colonize?

In summary, these principles are to:

- provide care that is ***regardful*** of culture.
- engage in *dialogue*—talk.
- ***ask*** what your clients want and ***how*** they want you to provide the services they want.
- be mindful of ***whose values*** are being valued.
- reflect on your own ***power and privilege*** and role in empowering others.
- ***process*** is more important than outcomes.
- continually ask yourself, 'are my ***actions empowering*** or disempowering?'
- examine the context for possible elements of *racism* or *discrimination*.
- *decolonize* your practice through examining language, assumptions, and behaviors.

There may be other principles you can add to the list above. However, even with just these few, there is a real opportunity to enhance the care experiences of culturally diverse Americans. Considering the enormous challenges of the current health and social status of sectors of our community, the role of health and human services professionals is an immensely important one.

Practice Strategies

We have discussed some practice principles and will now explore some practice strategies. For example, strengthening resilience encourages professionals to look for strengths and work with those. If a client needs to be more active, financial issues need to be considered as well as the environment that the person lives in. What interests and opportunities does the client have that can be used to develop an interest in and capacity to be more physically active?

'Deep listening' is a practice strategy that can build rapport and create an atmosphere that encourages communication. In the above example, a professional might respond by saying, 'That must be very hard', thereby acknowledging what was said, but then, 'how are you doing with that?' (thereby providing the opportunity for the client to elaborate).

De-Othering is the opposite of 'othering'. 'Othering' is when people treat 'others' who are different in some way from themselves as if they were in a different category. This is an 'I am this' and 'you are that' way of thinking and treating people. How do we know if we are 'othering'? We see evidence of 'othering' when people say things like, 'we don't do it that way, *we* do it like this', or 'how do *you people* ...', '*they* don't look after their health...' '*they* don't care...' Who are 'we' and who are 'you people' or 'them'? Look critically at the assumptions that are made in comments like these. De-Othering is about looking at similarities, as humans, rather than looking at differences or areas of separation between people or groups of people.

When we reflect on how the specific workplace that we work in, as well as the larger systems of health care and human services, influences how we work, what works, and what does not work, then we are in a better position to advocate for change. This can include building environments for change and being a part of that. It may include looking at the educational or employment influences on health and illness, not just at illness as something that needs to be diagnosed and treated.

Critical Thinking

> What is something that you could put into practice from what you have learned in this book?
>
> What have you learned about yourself while reflecting on some of the content of this book? Were there aspects that 'pushed your buttons' or possibly shifted a long-held belief?
>
> What if anything, might you do to enact cultural safety at a personal and organizational level?

The work of academics, researchers, and practitioners in taking cultural safety further is ongoing and there have been refinements and development of ideas and principles as we reflect on how this concept plays out in practice. Curtis et al. (2019) have turned their attention to the organizational level with their latest iteration of a cultural safety definition:

> Cultural safety requires healthcare professionals and their associated healthcare organisations to examine themselves and the potential impact of their own culture on clinical interactions and healthcare service delivery. This requires individual healthcare professionals and healthcare organisations to acknowledge and address their own biases, attitudes, assumptions, stereotypes, prejudices, structures and characteristics that may affect the quality of care provided. In doing so, cultural safety encompasses a critical consciousness where healthcare professionals and healthcare organisations engage in ongoing self-reflection and self-awareness and hold themselves accountable for providing culturally safe care, as defined by the patient and their communities, and as measured through progress towards achieving health equity. Cultural safety requires healthcare professionals and their associated healthcare organisations to influence healthcare to reduce bias and achieve equity within the workforce and working environment.

In operationalizing this approach to cultural safety, organizations (health professional training bodies, health care organizations, etc.) should begin with a self-review of the extent to which they meet expectations of cultural safety at a systemic and organizational level and identify an action plan for development. The following steps should also be considered by organizations and regulators to take a more comprehensive approach to cultural safety:

- Mandate evidence of engagement and transformation in cultural safety activities as a part of vocational training and professional development;
- Include evidence of cultural safety (of organisations and practitioners) as a requirement for accreditation and ongoing certification;
- Ensure that cultural safety is assessed by the systematic monitoring and assessment of inequities (in health workforce and health outcomes);
- Require cultural safety training and performance monitoring for staff, supervisors, and assessors;
- Acknowledge that cultural safety is an independent requirement that relates to, but is not restricted to, expectations for competency in ethnic or Indigenous health (Curtis et al., 2019).

Notice that in this definition, the emphasis has shifted from the individual to a shared responsibility with the health services to also examine their biases, attitudes, and barriers and to have a measurable outcome. But what are the structural barriers? Workforces have not really been discussed so far. How can the makeup of the workforce help or hinder the cultural safety of an organization? One of the common features of a culturally safe organization for clients is the opportunity to see someone of their own cultural background (age, gender, ability, ethnicity, etc.) in the service environment. How diverse then is the professional environment in your area? You might start looking to see how representative the workforce is of the people who access it. And if it is representative, in that there is diversity, where are these staff members in the organization? Are they at the client interface or are they in less visible roles, are they across all levels of the organization or only some? What will this say about the cultural safety of the organization? Racial or ethnic, gender and other representation have been addressed through certain strategies such as affirmative action, but that, too, has not been without controversy.

> Making It Local

> What other strategies and structural barriers need to be addressed to ensure an inclusive workforce? Look at each aspect of the recommendations and apply them to your own local health service or one you are familiar with. How does it measure up? If not, what would need to happen to make the organization culturally safe?

There has been some controversy in countries that have chosen to take up cultural safety as an approach to healthcare and resistance has come in many forms. If professionals talk about history and colonization they may be told, 'the past is the past; get over it'. If some people suggest that the 'helping professions' might actually harm their patients by continuing colonizing practices, they may be told that this perspective is 'outrageous'. If you were to tell a worker who is themselves struggling to put food on the table as bills mount up that they are privileged in their professional setting and that they have power, you may find that they are not very receptive to this point of view. Just like the debate that Black Lives Matter does not mean that other lives don't matter, cultural safety's focus on the need to decolonize, to examine and shift power, and to become aware of relative privilege, does not mean both cannot be true. Remember the diunital thinking we discussed earlier. You can be both powerless *and* powerful, depending on context. You can be oppressed, *and* you can also be a colonizer. You can be struggling, *and* you can be privileged. Cultural safety simply asks you to be regardful of these aspects of culture that have the potential to impact negatively on those you provide services or care to and, if anything, having experiences of both can give you something to draw upon to relate to and empathize with your clients.

Cultural Safety of Health and Human Service Professionals

We have talked almost exclusively about cultural safety for clients and communities, but we have not talked about what it means for health and human service professionals and other staff. Cultural safety is not and should not be a 'one-way street'. Those who provide services, you and your colleagues are also entitled to feel culturally safe in your workplace. You are no less entitled to provide service that does not demean or discriminate against you in the process. What has been our collective experience is that when you are able to provide culturally safe care, your safety, job satisfaction, and sense of achievement can be greater than anticipated.

Conclusion

A nation is only as strong as its most vulnerable populations. If any group is left behind on the basis of an aspect of who they are, (race, ethnicity, gender, sexuality, age, disability, religion, age, or any perceived difference) then that is a failure of the principles on which our country is founded. Health disparities and cultural issues are worthy of our collective attention by virtue of current failures to adequately meet the needs of various populations. As health and social service professionals, we can continue down a path that has seen certain members of the community excluded from the right to achieve optimal health, or we can use our practice to make a difference. If the experience of health and social care of one person is improved through a conscious effort to ensure cultural safety, then we will have achieved something significant.

References

Bassot, B. (2016). *The reflective practice guide: An interdisciplinary approach to critical reflection.* Routledge.

Browne, A. J., Varcoe, C., Smye, V., Reimer-Kirkham, S., Lynam, M. J., & Wong, S. (2009). Cultural safety and the challenges of translating critically oriented knowledge in practice. *Nursing Philosophy, 10*(3), 167–179.

Bulman, C., & Shutz, S. (2004). *Reflective practice in nursing* (3rd ed.). Boston: Blackwell.

Curtis, E., Jones, R., Tipene-Leach, D., Curtis, W., Belinda, L., Sarah-Jane, P., & Papaarangi, R. (2019). Why cultural safety rather than cultural competency is required to achieve health equity: A literature review and recommended definition. *International Journal of Equity in Health, 18*, 174. https://doi.org/10.1186/s12939-019-1082-3.

Elliot, M. (2004). *Reflective thinking: Turning a critical incident into a topic for research*. https://www.nursingtimes.net/clinical-archive/leadership/reflective-thinking-turning-a-critical-incident-into-a-topic-for-research-01-01-2004/.

Frankel, R., & Stein, T. (1999). Getting the most out of the clinical encounter: The four habits model. *The Permanente Journal, 3*, 79–88.

Freire, P. (1972). *Pedagogy of the oppressed*. Penguin.

Gabb, D., & McDermott, D. (2007). What do Indigenous experiences and perspectives mean for transcultural mental health? Towards a new model of transcultural teaching for health professionals. In R. Ranzijn, K. McConnochie & W. Nolan (Eds.), *Psychology and indigenous Australians—Teaching, practice and theory*. Cambridge Scholars Publishing.

Grant, J., & Guerin, P. (2018). Mixed and misunderstandings: An exploration of the meaning of racism with maternal, child and family health nurses in South Australia. *Journal of Advanced Nursing*. https://doi.org/10.1111/jan.13789.

Howatson-Jones, L. (2016). *Reflective practice in nursing* (3rd ed.). Sage.

Johns, C. (Ed.). (2017). *Becoming a reflective practitioner* (5th Ed.) Wiley-Blackwell.

Johns, C., & Freshwater, D. (2005). *Transforming nursing through reflective practice* (2nd ed.). Wiley-Blackwell.

McEldowney, R., Richardson, F., Turia, D., Laracy, K., Scott, W., & MacDonald, S. (2006). *Opening our eyes—Shifting our thinking. The process of teaching and learning about reflection in cultural safety education and practice: An evaluation study*. Kapiti Print Media Ltd, Victoria University of Wellington and Whitireia Community Polytechnic.

Mezirow, J. (1991). *Transformative dimensions of adult learning*. Jossey-Bass.

Oelke, N. D., Thurston, W. E., & Arthur, N. (2013). Intersections between interprofessional practice, cultural competency and primary healthcare. *Journal of Interprofessional Care, 27*(5), 367–372. https://doi.org/10.3109/13561820.2013.785502. Epub 2013 May 17. PMID: 23683058.

Ramsden, I. (2002). *Cultural Safety and Nursing Education in Aotearoa and Te Waipounamu*. Wellington: University of Wellington.

Rosen, D., McCall, J., & Goodkind, S. (2017). Teaching critical self-reflection through the lens of cultural humility: An assignment in a social work diversity course. *Social Work Education, 36*(3), 289–298. https://doi.org/10.1080/02615479.2017.1287260.

Schön, D. (1983). *The reflective practitioner: How professionals think in action.* Temple Smith.

Wepa, D. (Ed.). (2015). *Cultural Safety in Aotearoa New Zealand* (2nd ed.). Cambridge: Cambridge University Press. https://doi.org/10.1017/CBO9781316151136.

Index

A
African American 13, 15, 26, 103, 148
Aging 177, 191, 209, 210
Alcoholism 117, 118
American Indian. *See* Native American/Alaska Native
Anti-racism 94, 151
Asian 13, 15, 28, 103, 129, 178, 179, 185, 209, 210
Assimilation 28, 103, 108, 269, 272–274
Australia 6, 47, 56, 58, 131, 261–264, 266, 271–277, 279, 280, 282–284

B
Biomedical model 65, 66, 69, 70, 72, 167

Biopsychosocial model 70
Black American 28, 97, 106, 150, 155, 170, 184, 192, 230

C
Canada 6, 47, 56, 131, 150, 261, 262, 264–266, 269, 274–280, 282–284
Capacity 12, 19, 90, 121, 151, 217–219, 221, 224–227, 230, 232–234, 237, 280, 300
Chronic diseases 20, 26, 67, 171, 197–199, 209, 257
Colonization 2, 8, 14, 19–22, 28, 30, 42, 56, 90, 91, 94–98, 107, 111, 140, 198, 224, 230, 235, 261–265, 271, 274, 275, 278, 279, 281, 283, 303

Community-based participatory research 113
Cultural awareness 26, 30, 31, 33, 38, 48, 51–53, 55, 166
Cultural competence 7, 26, 30–32, 34, 35, 39
Cultural humility 27, 35, 39
Cultural safety 2, 4–7, 10, 19–23, 26, 27, 29–32, 37, 38, 40–42, 45–53, 55–59, 62, 66, 67, 74, 80–82, 84, 87, 107, 108, 111, 115, 127, 128, 130, 133, 142, 154, 162, 192, 203, 210, 212, 217–219, 226, 235, 237, 239, 240, 245, 250, 251, 253, 257, 259, 281, 283, 288, 291–294, 296, 298, 301–304
Cultural sensitivity 26, 31, 39, 53, 55, 235
Culture 2, 4, 7, 9, 11, 13, 15, 16, 19, 21, 23, 25–36, 38, 39, 41, 42, 46–53, 55, 56, 61, 66, 71, 77, 85, 86, 101, 104, 107, 108, 117, 118, 127–129, 137, 138, 141, 142, 149–151, 162, 165, 171, 174, 180, 186, 192, 198, 206, 207, 209–211, 224, 229, 234, 235, 240, 241, 245, 253, 254, 259, 262, 266, 272, 279, 281, 287, 288, 293, 294, 299, 301, 303
Culture responsiveness 27, 36

D

Decolonize 2, 9, 21, 22, 38, 42, 48, 61, 111, 239, 240, 282, 287, 299, 303

Diabetes 5, 20, 26, 68, 97, 192, 197–199, 256
Dichotomous 116–118, 127, 129
Disability 7, 29, 67, 80, 100, 101, 125, 170, 172, 175, 186, 191, 192, 194, 211, 212, 226, 304
Discrimination 4, 30, 37, 55, 71, 128, 137, 138, 142, 148–151, 153–156, 162, 193, 200, 212, 292, 299
Diunital 116–118, 127, 129, 162, 303
Doctrine of Discovery 91, 93, 94, 99
Drug addiction 118

E

Education 26, 36, 47, 59, 70, 73, 82, 85, 137–140, 142–144, 146, 147, 151, 168, 172, 180, 193, 197–200, 203, 220, 230, 243, 289
Employment 17, 82, 101, 137–140, 144, 146, 168, 172, 175, 193, 254, 300
Epidemiology 165, 166, 171
Epistemology 116
Equality 3, 152, 153
Equity 41, 47, 48, 50, 79, 138, 139, 151–153, 155, 194, 196, 224, 261, 270, 293, 301
Ethics 124
Ethnicity 2, 4, 9, 12–14, 16, 26, 28, 46, 102, 105, 119, 143, 149, 150, 171, 184, 185, 192, 202, 205, 211, 226, 277, 289, 297, 302, 304

F

Female circumcision/Female genital mutilation (FGM) 127–131

H

Health disparities 2, 32, 126, 148, 152, 175, 196, 203, 271, 304
HIV 200
Homelessness 147
Housing 20, 73, 77, 82, 137–140, 144, 146, 147, 161, 168, 180, 193, 199

I

Identity 7, 9–11, 14, 15, 17, 18, 22, 29, 30, 36, 41, 50, 53, 101–105, 109, 111, 118, 137, 141, 142, 146, 149, 151, 159, 162, 171, 172, 174, 180, 181, 184–186, 192, 199, 205, 224, 229, 243, 277, 278, 298
Indigenous 6, 8, 14, 15, 20, 46–48, 56, 58, 67–69, 71, 74, 77, 79, 85, 91–93, 95, 96, 99, 100, 105, 108, 115, 139, 155, 181, 185, 186, 192, 200, 209, 228, 230, 231, 261–267, 269, 271–283, 293, 302
Infant health 202, 203
Infectious disease 191, 200, 201
Initialism 9

L

LGBTQIAA (LGBT, LGBTQ) xii, 9, 62, 79, 101
Liberation 3, 152, 281

M

Maternal health 197, 202, 203
Mental health 10, 20, 118, 133, 191, 206–208, 229, 233
Meritocracy 145
MOVE bombing 106

N

Native American/Alaska Native 13, 14, 26, 28, 93, 96, 103, 104, 108–110, 155, 172–174, 178, 184, 185, 219, 274, 276, 277
Native Hawaiian 13, 103, 177–179, 185
New Zealand 6, 29, 30, 47, 55–59, 131, 261, 262, 264, 266, 270, 271, 274, 276–284
Nuremberg code 125

O

Opioid epidemic 205
Othering 4, 55, 212, 300

P

Pacific Islander 13, 103, 177, 179, 185
Parasitic disease 200, 201
Prevention 20, 73, 77, 81, 86, 193, 197, 255
Primary health care (PHC) 74–84, 87, 217

R

Race 2, 4, 9, 12–14, 26, 28, 46, 102, 105, 118, 119, 143, 149,

150, 154, 167, 171, 177, 184, 185, 192, 202, 261, 265, 273, 297, 304
Racism 4, 12, 30, 55, 124, 137, 138, 142, 148–151, 154–156, 162, 299
Randomized control trials 71
Regardful 62, 142, 282, 287, 294, 303
Research 4, 12, 36, 38, 62, 70–72, 78, 106, 113–116, 121–127, 129, 132, 133, 142, 176, 202, 203, 220, 228, 241, 242, 254, 291, 298
Resilience 19, 86, 142, 217–221, 223, 224, 226–228, 230, 233, 234, 300

S
Social determinants of health (SDoH) 20, 73, 78, 138–140, 194, 196, 209
Social model 2, 69, 70, 73
Socio-economic status/Social and economic status (SES) 26, 70, 138, 141
Substance use 203

T
Terra nullius 93, 94, 98, 99, 272
Tulsa Massacre 106
Tuskegee syphilis study 124

W
Wealth 98, 138, 144–146
Worldview 8, 31, 56, 62, 69, 86, 94, 102, 111, 113, 115–118, 131–133, 139, 178, 180, 199, 206, 207, 239, 242, 256

The manufacturer's authorised representative in the EU is Springer Nature Customer Service Centre GmbH, Europaplatz 3, 69115 Heidelberg, Germany. If you have any concerns regarding our products, please contact ProductSafety@springernature.com

Printed and bound by CPI Group (UK) Ltd, Croydon, CR0 4YY

25/03/2026

02078175-0005